Corinne Bak

MANUAL OF

MW01045480

Already published in the Manuals series

Cardiology *K. Dawkins*
Chest Medicine *J. E. Stark, J. M. Shneerson, T. Higenbottam, C. D.R. Flower*
Clinical Blood Transfusion *M. Brozović, B. Brozović*
Gynaecology *T. R. Varma*
Haematology *A. S. J. Baughan. A. S. B. Hughes, K. G. Patterson, L. Stirling*
Paediatric Gastroenterology *J. H. Tripp, D. C. A. Candy*
Renal Disease *C. B. Brown*
Rheumatology *J. M. H. Moll*

Forthcoming volumes

Accident and Emergency Medicine *S. Lord*
Geriatric Medicine *A. Exton-Smith, T. Van der Cammen*
Intensive Care Medicine *K. Hillman*
Medical Procedures *M. J. Ford, C. E. Robertson, J. F. Munro*
Neonatal Intensive Care *A. R. Wilkinson*
Neonatal Medicine *D. Harvey, M. Cummins*
Paediatrics *J. Hambleton*

MANUAL OF GASTRO-ENTEROLOGY

B. T. Cooper BSc MD MRCP
Consultant Gastroenterologist
Dudley Road Hospital
Birmingham

M. J. Hall MB MSc MRCP
Lecturer in Medicine
University Department of Medicine
Bristol Royal Infirmary

R. E. Barry BSc MD FRCP
Consultant Senior Lecturer in Medicine
University Department of Medicine
Bristol Royal Infirmary
Bristol UK

Foreword by
A. E. Read MD FRCP
Professor of Medicine
University of Bristol

Churchill Livingstone ▦

EDINBURGH LONDON MELBOURNE AND NEW YORK 1987

CHURCHILL LIVINGSTONE
Medical Division of Longman Group UK Limited

Distributed in the United States of America by Churchill Livingstone Inc., 1560 Broadway, New York, N.Y. 10036, and by associated companies, branches and representatives throughout the world.

© Longman Group UK Limited 1987

All rights reserved. No part of this publication may be reproduced, stored in a retrieval system, or transmitted in any form or by any means, electronic, mechanical, photocopying, recording or otherwise, without the prior permission of the publishers (Churchill Livingstone, Robert Stevenson House, 1–3 Baxter's Place, Leith Walk, Edinburgh EH1 3AF).

First published 1987

ISBN 0 443 02957 1

British Library Cataloguing in Publication Data
Cooper, B. T.
    Manual of gastroenterology.
    1. Gastrointestinal system — Diseases —
    Diagnosis
    I. Title   II. Hall, M. J.   III. Barry, R. E.
    616.3'3075   RC803

Library of Congress Cataloging in Publication Data
Cooper, B. T.
    Manual of gastroenterology.
    (Manual series)
    Includes index.
    1. Gastrointestinal system — Diseases — Handbooks,
manuals, etc.   I. Hall, M. J. (Michael Joseph)
II. Barry, R. E.   III. Title. [DNLM: 1. Gastro-
intestinal Diseases.   WI 100 C776m]
RC801.C664   1986   616.3'3   86–26920

Produced by Longman Singapore Publishers (Pte) Ltd.
Printed in Singapore.

FOREWORD

There is no shortage of textbooks on gastroenterology, so one has to look rather critically at any new book to see how it may complement the many others. There is in any case a variety of types of gastroenterology textbook, ranging from the weighty, well-referenced and often outdated large textbook, to the pocket synopsis used as a practical guide or exam crammer. This book belongs amongst the last group but it is outstanding amongst them in the amount of information it contains. The writers, who are all gastroenterological experts with plenty of experience, commonsense, and who are fully aware of the growing points of their subject, have written an essentially brief but pragmatic and useful account of the subject.

The first part of the book provides details of the major causes of gastrointestinal symptoms, whilst the second describes the common gastrointestinal disorders including their investigation and treatment. Of necessity the number of diseases described is limited and sometimes brief, but little of importance has been left out — further, diseases of the pancreas, liver and biliary tree are also included in addition to those of the alimentary canal. Wisely there is also a section on nutritional support as these techniques are so essential for good gastroenterological practice.

Junior staff in this country often rotate through several specialties over the course of a one or two year appointment. A book like this should soon allow them to be conversant with the basic facts concerning the clinical world of gastroenterology, and its reading either completely or piecemeal would not take too long.

I therefore view this book as a valuable contribution to gastroenterology — not only for the expert for whom it makes a brief and readable summary but also for the stranger to the subject, be he or she a clinical student, houseman or more senior member of the hospital staff.

I wish it well; it deserves to do so.

1987   A. E. R.

PREFACE

The aim of this book is to give practical advice on the diagnosis, management and treatment of the common and important gastroenterological (including hepatological) diseases. It is not designed to be a comprehensive mini-textbook of gastroenterology and, therefore, certain aspects — particularly on the aetiology, epidemiology and pathology of gastrointestinal disease — are only considered in the briefest detail and rare diseases are not included. The book is aimed primarily at physicians and therefore surgical aspects are only mentioned where they are relevant to medical practice. There are three sections — on assessment of symptoms, diagnosis and treatment of specific disorders, and practical clinical nutrition as applied to gastrointestinal disease. We feel that nutrition is a particularly important aspect of modern gastroenterological practice and one that is often ignored or given little space in standard textbooks on gastroenterological disease. The book is designed to be small and pocket sized and the text is telegrammatic and didactic so that useful practical information can be obtained easily. We are aware that this format allows no room for discussion of the many controversial areas in modern gastroenterology. We make no apology for putting forward our own views in the belief that they have served us well and provide a helpful and effective practical approach to the various problems. However, when controversy exists, we have indicated as much in the text.

This book is directed principally at registrars (or residents) in gastroenterological units, however other physicians who have only an occasional exposure to patients with gastroenterological disorders may find it useful. The book will also be valuable to house staff and nursing staff who look after patients with gastroenterological problems and to surgical staff who often deal with medical gastroenterological problems. Students or trained gastroenterologists may find aspects of the book helpful and interesting.

We would like to thank Andrew Stevenson of Churchill Livingstone for suggesting the book and for encouraging us to write it. Finally, we would like to thank our colleagues for the helpful discussion clarifying various aspects of gastroenterological practice.

1987

B. T.C.
M. J. H.
R. E. B.

CONTENTS

ABBREVIATIONS

AAA	Aromatic amino acids
AMA	Anti-mitochondrial antibodies
ANF	Antinuclear factor
Anti-HBc	Antibody to hepatitis B core antigen
Anti-HBs	Antibody to hepatitis B surface antigen
AST	Aspartate aminotransferase
BCAA	Branched chain amino acid
bd	L. *bis die*, twice a day
BP	Blood pressure
BIDA	Parabutyl iminodiacetate
CT	Computerized tomography
CVP	Central venous pressure
DU	Duodenal ulcer
DVT	Deep venous thrombosis
ECG	Electrocardiogram
EEG	Electroencephalogram
ERCP	Endoscopic retrograde cholangiopancreatography
ESR	Erythrocyte sedimentation rate
FBC	Full blood count
GI	Gastrointestinal
γGT	Gamma glutamyl transferase
GU	Gastric ulcer
H_2	Cellular receptor site for histamine responsible for the stimulation of gastric secretion
HAV	Hepatitis A virus
HBV	Hepatitis B virus
HBcAg	Hepatitis B core antigen
HBeAg	Hepatitis B 'e' antigen
HBsAg	Hepatitis B surface antigen
H & E staining	Haematoxylin and eosin
HCAT	23-selena-25-homocholyl taurine
IBD	Inflammatory bowel disease
IBS	Irritable bowel syndrome
ITU	Intensive therapy unit
IVC	Intravenous cholangiography
JVP	Jugular venous pressure

LOS	Lower oesophageal sphincter
MCV	Mean corpuscular volume
MSU	Midstream urine
nocte	L. *nocte*, at night
PAS	Periodic acid Schiff
PBC	Primary biliary cirrhosis
PCV	Packed cell volume
PR	Per rectum
PTC	Percutaneous transhepatic cholangiography
qds	L. *Quater die sumendum*, to be taken four times a day
SBE	Subacute bacterial (infective) endocarditis
SI	Small intestine
SMA	Smooth muscle antibodies
TB	Tubercle bacillus
tds	L. *ter die sumendum*, to be taken three times a day
TIBC	Total iron binding capacity
UC	ulcerative colitis
U/S	Ultrasound scan
VIP	Vasoactive intestinal peptide
WCC	White cell count

PART ONE
Symptoms

1. DYSPHAGIA, OTHER OESOPHAGEAL SYMPTOMS, EPIGASTRIC PAIN AND DYSPEPSIA

DYSPHAGIA

This is difficulty in swallowing. The patient usually complains of food sticking somewhere between mouth and stomach. It is an important symptom that should never be dismissed.

Causes of dysphagia

Oropharyngeal dysphagia

 Striated muscle disorders — neurological, myopathic
 Inflammatory lesions of mouth, pharynx and larynx
 Tumours of larynx and pharynx
 Retropharyngeal abscess
 Paterson–Kelly (Plummer–Vinson) syndrome
 Zenker's diverticulum (pharyngeal pouch)
 Goitre
 (Globus hystericus — not a true dysphagia because the patient complains of a continuous lump in the throat)

Oesophageal dysphagia

Intraoesophageal disease

 Benign stricture — reflux oesophagitis, corrosive oesophagitis, trauma
 Carcinoma
 Rings and webs
 Motor disorders — achalasia, diffuse spasm, systemic sclerosis

Extrinsic pressure

 Mediastinal nodes or tumours
 Aneurysm
 Large left atrium
 Dysphagia lusoria (compression of oesophagus by anomalous right subclavian artery (or other major vessel)
 Paraoesophageal (rolling) hiatal hernia

Important questions

1. What is the level of the dysphagia? — The patient usually gives a reliable indication of the level of the obstruction but occasionally a low stricture will cause the patient to complain of high dysphagia.
2. What is the length of history? — It may be years (e.g achalasia) or only a few weeks or months (e.g. carcinoma).
3. Is the dysphagia intermittent (as in achalasia or spasm) or persistent (as in carcinoma)?
4. Is it progressive (as in carcinoma) non-progressive (as in achalasia or spasm) or very slowly progressive (as in benign stricture)?
5. How severe is it? This is assessed by the nature of food obstruction — in severe dysphagia the patient may have symptoms after drinking liquids
6. What associated features are present? — A previous history of gastro-oesophageal reflux suggests a peptic stricture; pain on swallowing may be seen in diffuse spasm or carcinoma; coughing after swallowing is common with a pharyngeal pouch; regurgitation immediately after swallowing is a feature of any severe dysphagia, especially carcinoma and achalasia.

Investigations

Oropharyngeal dysphagia

1. Barium swallow — this is especially useful if combined with cineradiography to assess the act of swallowing.
2. Inspection of pharynx, laryngoscopy and inspection of the upper oesophagus with fibreoptic oesophagoscope.

Oesophageal dysphagia

1. Barium swallow — this is a mandatory investigation. If story is good but the barium swallow appears normal, subtle degrees of obstruction may be shown by getting the patient to swallow a piece of bread or marshmallow soaked in barium.
2. Fibreoptic oesophagoscopy — this allows inspection of the oesophagus with biopsy and brush cytology of any lesion. The presence of oesophageal obstruction increases the risk of perforating the oesophagus with the endoscope, so a barium swallow is necessary before proceeding to endoscopy. Endoscopy may be contraindicated in the presence of a pharyngeal pouch.

OTHER OESOPHAGEAL SYMPTOMS

Heartburn (pyrosis)
Retrosternal burning, especially after drinking hot liquids, on bending or on lying flat; it is a most important symptom of gastro-oesophageal reflux.

Regurgitation
Effortless bringing up of gastric contents on bending or lying. It is a cardinal symptom of gastro-oesophageal reflux. It is often associated with heartburn. It must be distinguished from vomiting by close questioning as some patients refer to it as vomiting. Regurgitation immediately after swallowing may be seen in severe dysphagia of any cause.

Oesophageal pain
Painful swallowing (odynophagia) may be seen in gastro-oesophageal reflux, oesophageal carcinoma, ulcer or diffuse spasm. Oesophageal colic is not common and is seen characteristically in diffuse spasm, early in the course of achalasia and occasionally in gastro-oesophageal reflux. Oesophageal pain may be very severe and may mimic myocardial pain, even to the extent of radiating down the arm and being aggravated or initiated by exertion.

Dyspepsia
Post prandial epigastric discomfort and bloating may be described by patients with gastro-oesophageal reflux.

Symptoms of pulmonary aspiration
Coughing, especially at night, nocturnal asthma or dyspnoea, recurrent bronchitis or pneumonia may be seen over a long period in patients with achalasia or gastro-oesophageal reflux, and over a shorter period in patients with severe dysphagia of any cause. Patients with carcinoma may have pulmonary symptoms because they develop a carcinomatous tracheo–oesophageal fistula.

Waterbrash
This confusing term should be restricted to the filling of the mouth with clear fluid (probably saliva) which is seen in patients with peptic ulcer as well as those with gastro-oesophageal reflux.

EPIGASTRIC PAIN AND DYSPEPSIA

Pain felt in the epigastrium may be described as indigestion or even chest pain by the patient. Indigestion (or dyspepsia) is a confusing term and patients should be closely questioned as to what they mean by it. Indigestion (or dyspepsia) is upper abdominal discomfort, heaviness or early satiety related to eating. Heartburn, retrosternal chest pain, regurgitation and flatulence may also be described as indigestion by patients.

Causes of epigastric pain and dyspepsia

Peptic ulceration — acute or chronic
Gastritis
Oesophagitis
Gastric carcinoma
Pancreatitis — acute or chronic
Pancreatic carcinoma
Gall bladder disease
Portal hypertension
Irritable bowel syndrome
Non-ulcer dyspepsia

Rarer causes of epigastric pain: tabes dorsalis, root pain, diabetic ketoacidosis, aortic aneurysm, polycythaemia, mesenteric angina, coeliac axis compression syndrome, Menetrier's disease.

N.B. Dyspepsia may be caused by non GI disorders, e.g. uraemia, cardiac failure, TB, neoplasia.

Important questions

1. What is the site, character, radiation, frequency, duration, periodicity, severity, mode of onset and cessation of the pain?
2. Are there any aggravating or relieving factors such as antacids, vomiting, posture, defaecation, food?
3. Are there any associated symptoms such as nausea, vomiting, etc.?
4. Does the pain radiate through to the back as in posterior wall chronic DU, chronic pancreatitis or pancreatic carcinoma?
5. Has the character of long standing dyspepsia or epigastric pain changed? This suggests gastric carcinoma.
6. Does the pain immediately follow eating and/or is it relieved by vomiting? This suggests gastritis, gastric ulcer or oesophagitis.
7. Does the pain come on 0.5–1 hour after food or longer? This suggests duodenal ulcer, gastric outflow obstruction, chronic pancreatitis, mesenteric angina.
8. Are the symptoms relieved by food as with duodenal ulcer?
9. Does the pain awake the patient in the early hours of the morning? This suggests duodenal ulcer or oesophagitis.
10. Is the pain constant as in pancreatic or gastric carcinoma or mesenteric ischaemia?
11. Can the site of the pain be localised by one finger? The 'pointing sign' is said to be a feature of duodenal ulceration.

Investigations

1. Full blood count.
2. Upper GI endoscopy — first choice.
3. Barium meal — if endoscopy is unavailable or unhelpful.
4. Other investigations (e.g. ultrasound, cholecystogram, ERCP, etc.) may be indicated if endoscopy is negative and/or history and examination suggest another cause.

2. ANOREXIA, WEIGHT LOSS AND VOMITING

ANOREXIA

Causes of anorexia

Gastrointestinal disease
Infection
Malignancy
Heart failure
Respiratory failure
Metabolic disorders e.g. uraemia, hypercalcaemia
Endocrine disease e.g. Addison's disease, hypopituitarism,
   hyperparathyroidism
Psychiatric disorders e.g. depression, anxiety, anorexia nervosa
Drugs, e.g. digoxin
Toxins, e.g. alcohol

Important questions

These should differentiate anorexia from early satiety, food intolerance
and sitophobia (fear of eating which may be seen in oesophagitis, gastric
ulcer, partial small intestinal obstruction, mesenteric angina) and pay
attention to drugs being taken.

Investigations

Depend on findings after full history and examination.

WEIGHT LOSS

Significant weight loss (5% or more of body weight) is an important
symptom which frequently indicates organic disease. Weight loss results
from decreased food intake, increased tissue catabolism or loss of
calories (e.g. in faeces or urine).

Causes of weight loss

Gastrointestinal disease — especially oesophageal and gastric disorders, malabsorption, inflammatory bowel disease, intestinal obstruction, malignancy

Malignancy — any site

Diabetes mellitus

Thyrotoxicosis

Infection, e.g. TB, infective endocarditis

Infestations

Uraemia

Cardiac failure

Respiratory failure

Dehydration

Diuretic therapy

Drugs, smoking, alcohol

Psychiatric disorders, e.g. anorexia nervosa, depression, schizophrenia

Important questions

1. Has the patient been on a weight reducing diet or on an inadequate diet?
2. Is the weight loss occurring in spite of a good appetite as in malabsorption, diabetes or thyrotoxicosis?
3. Is the weight loss associated with anorexia as in oesophageal or gastric disease, uraemia, infection, cardiac failure or malignancy?

Investigations

1. Full history and examination will often reveal the likely cause or areas to be investigated.
2. Minimal investigations are:
   a. Full blood count, ESR, blood urea, serum creatinine and electrolytes
   b. Liver function tests, blood sugar, thyroid function tests.
   c. Urinalysis and culture
   d. Chest X-ray

VOMITING

This symptom always needs to be taken seriously because of the risk of metabolic consequences even if the cause may be trivial. Nausea usually but not always precedes it.

Causes of vomiting

Gastrointestinal disease

Stomach	— ulcer	
	carcinoma	
	gastritis	
	obstruction	
	post-gastrectomy	
	vagotomy	
	gastric neuropathy e.g. diabetes	
Pylorus	— obstruction	
	ulcer	
Duodenum	— obstruction	
	ulcer	
Intestine	— obstruction	
	infarction	
	inflammation — idiopathic, infective	

      Pancreatitis
      Cholecystitis
      Appendicitis
      Peritonitis

Liver disease
      Acute hepatitis
      Acute hepatic failure

Infections, e.g. viral, urinary tract

Metabolic disorders
      Uraemia
      Ketoacidosis
      Hypercalcaemia
      Addisonian crisis

Neurological disorders
      Meningitis
      Migraine
      Raised intracranial pressure
      Meniere's disease

Cardiovascular disorders
      Acute myocardial infarction
      Shock
      Acute hypertension

Psychological disorders
      Psychogenic vomiting
      Anorexia nervosa

Drugs e.g. opiates, digoxin, anti- metabolites

Toxins e.g. alcohol

Pregnancy

General anaesthesia

Radiotherapy

Motion sickness

Risks of vomiting

1. Metabolic— Dehydration
   Electrolyte depletion (Na^+, K^+)
   Metabolic alkalosis (loss of H^+)
2. Mendelson's syndrome (aspiration pneumonitis)
3. Boerhaave's syndrome (spontaneous rupture of the oesophagus)
4. Mallory-Weiss syndrome (mucosal tear at cardia)

Important questions

1. Is the patient actually vomiting? Regurgitation secondary to gastro-oesophageal reflux and symptoms from oesophageal stricture or oesophageal diverticulum may be described as vomiting.
2. Is the vomiting preceded by nausea? Vomiting of raised intracranial pressure and pyloric stenosis are sometimes not preceded by nausea.
3. Does vomiting follow meals? This is a feature of psychogenic vomiting and pyloric channel ulcer and sometimes of gastric ulcer and gastritis.
4. What time does the vomiting occur? Early morning vomiting is a feature of pregnancy, alcoholism, uraemia and bilious vomiting after partial gastrectomy.
5. Does vomiting relieve associated abdominal pain? This suggests gastric ulcer.
6. What are the contents of the vomitus? Note whether it contains gastric secretions alone or blood, coffee grounds, food, bile, or 'faecal' material. If food eaten more than 12 hours previously is recognised, this suggests gastric outflow obstruction or delayed gastric emptying. 'Faecal' vomiting suggests intestinal obstruction or infarction.
7. Is the vomitus particularly offensive to smell? If so it suggests gastric outflow obstruction or diabetic gastric neuropathy.
8. Is the vomiting projectile? This is difficult to define but can be a feature of raised intracranial pressure and occasionally pyloric stenosis. However it is not restricted to these disorders.
9. What drugs are being taken?

Investigations

1. Blood electrolytes, urea, sugar, calcium, liver function tests and acid-base studies
2. Urinalysis and culture
3. Plain abdominal X-ray
4. Barium meal and/or upper GI endoscopy
5. Other investigations will be determined by the history and physical findings, e.g. pregnancy test, CT scan of the brain

3. GASTROINTESTINAL BLEEDING, ABDOMINAL SWELLING AND ASCITES

GASTROINTESTINAL BLEEDING

This important symptom may be overt with haematemesis, melaena or fresh blood per rectum or occult with faeces positive for blood on chemical testing and/or with iron deficiency anaemia.

Causes of gastrointestinal bleeding

Oesophagus
- Reflux oesophagitis
- Drug-induced or corrosive oesophagitis
- Candidal oesophagitis
- Varices
- Carcinoma
- Mallory-Weiss tear
- Achalasia (rare)

Stomach
- Gastritis and erosions, e.g. drug-induced
- Ulcer
- Carcinoma
- Other tumours (rare)
- Varices (rare)
- Menetrier's disease (rare)

Duodenum
- Ulcer
- Diverticulum
- Ampullary carcinoma
- Duodenal carcinoma (rare)
- Aorto-duodenal fistula (rare)
- Haemobilia (rare)
- Pancreatic carcinoma (rare)
- Acute pancreatitis (rare)

Small intestine (most relatively rare)
- Meckel's diverticulum
- Ulceration e.g. Crohn's disease, non-specific enteritis

       Carcinoma
       Lymphoma
       Jejunal diverticulosis
       Ischaemia
       Intussusception
       Infestation e.g. Hookworm (rare in UK; common worldwide)
Large intestine
       Anal disorders e.g. haemorrhoids
       Carcinoma
       Polyp
       Rectal ulcer
       Colitis — idiopathic
                 infective
                 ischaemic
       Diverticular disease
       Endometriosis (rare)
       Varices (rare)
Anywhere in GI tract (most are rare)
       Bleeding disorders
       Anticoagulant therapy
       Angiodysplasia   } relatively common
       Radiation damage
       Hereditary haemorrhagic
         telangiectasia
       Other vascular anomalies e.g. haemangioma, vasculitis
           Henoch-Schönlein purpura
           Polyarteritis nodosa
           Systemic lupus erythematosus
       Connective tissue disorders
           Pseudoxanthoma elasticum
           Ehlers–Danlos syndrome
       Systemic sclerosis
       Intestinal polyposis syndromes

   Oesophageal and gastric causes of brisk bleeding are likely to lead to
haematemesis whereas bleeding from the duodenum or more distally in
the GI tract is more likely to cause melaena. If blood has remained long
enough in the stomach, the patient will vomit blood altered by HCl, i.e.
'coffee grounds'. Any severe proximal GI bleed will cause haematemesis
and melaena. If colonic transit is slow, bleeding from the proximal colon
causes melaena. Fresh blood per rectum suggests distal large bowel
bleeding. Blood covering the stool or following the stool suggests
anorectal bleeding but blood mixed with the stool suggests more
proximal colonic bleeding. However, torrential haemorrhage from any
site in the GI tract may cause fresh blood per rectum. Any of the lesions
listed can cause occult GI blood loss. Common causes are peptic ulcer,

gastritis, reflux oesophagitis, haemorrhoids, neoplasms, diverticular disease and inflammatory bowel disease. Do not forget to consider malabsorption in the patient with diarrhoea and iron deficiency especially if faecal occult blood tests are negative.

Important questions

1. Has the patient really had a haematemesis? Epistaxis and haemoptysis can be confused with or difficult to differentiate from haematemesis.
2. Has the patient really had melaena? Iron or bismuth containing medications and recent ingestion of liquorice, liver or black puddings, etc. can cause black stools. Excessive beetroot ingestion can cause red stools.
3. Has the patient had any associated or preceding symptoms of GI disease — e.g. dysphagia, dyspepsia, abdominal pain, vomiting, retching, abnormal bowel habit, jaundice?
4. What drugs has the patient taken? Especially important are aspirin, non-steroidal anti-inflammatory drugs, corticosteroids, anticoagulants. Enquire about and check contents of any proprietary medication taken.
5. How much alcohol does the patient drink?
6. Has the patient bled from the GI tract before?
7. Is there a history of bleeding from other sites, post-operative bleeding or easy bruising?
8. Has the patient had gastrointestinal surgery or irradiation?
9. Is there a family history of bleeding?

Investigations

In all cases

1. Rectal examination and faecal occult blood testing as part of the physical examination
2. Full blood count, ESR, prothrombin time
3. Blood urea, electrolytes, liver function tests

In suspected upper GI tract bleeding

1. Upper GI endoscopy — preferably within 12 hours of admission if the patient has had haematemesis or melaena.
2. Barium meal — only indicated if endoscopy is unavailable or is unhelpful. Barium will obscure view for angiography.
3. Difficult cases:
   a. Full coagulation screen
   b. Red cell isotope scan
   c. Angiography
   d. Emergency laparotomy if severe haemorrhage with no obvious cause of if there is not time for angiography.

In suspected lower intestinal bleeding

1. Sigmoidoscopy — preferably with the flexible fibreoptic sigmoidoscope
2. Colonoscopy
3. Barium enema — if endoscopy not available; barium will obscure angiographic pictures
4. Difficult cases —
   a. Full coagulation screen
   b. Red cell isotope scan
   c. Angiography.

Occult GI bleeding

1. Full coagulation screen.
2. Investigate upper GI tract and rectum and colon.
3. Investigate small bowel —
   a. Barium follow through
   b. Red cell isotope scan
   c. Meckel's scan
   d. Angiography.
4. Laparotomy — only in last resort if all other tests are negative and patient has significant blood loss.

ABDOMINAL SWELLING

Causes of abdominal swelling

Fat — most frequent cause
Aerophagy and functional (non-ulcer) dyspepsia
Irritable bowel syndrome (IBS)
Intestinal obstruction
Malabsorption
Toxic dilatation of the colon
Ascites
Constipation
Abdominal masses, e.g. tumours, enlarged liver, spleen
Cysts — pancreatic, ovarian
Enlarged bladder
Pregnant uterus

N.B. Most bowel related abdominal swelling is caused by flatus

Important questions

1. Is the swelling intermittent or persistent? The former is seen in IBS, aerophagy, malabsorption, partial obstruction. In IBS or aerophagy there is often little objective evidence of swelling and the patient may refer to early satiety and bloating as abdominal swelling. Persistent swelling suggests

ascites, abdominal cysts, masses or fat and is associated with weight increase and the need for clothes of increasing girth.
2. Is the swelling worse after eating? This suggests bowel related swelling or aerophagy; patients may report the need to loosen clothes after eating.
3. Is the swelling associated with abdominal rumbling? Suggests malabsorption, obstruction or occasionally irritable bowel syndrome.
4. Is the swelling eased by passing flatus? Common in aerophagy and IBS.
5. Is the swelling associated with the recent occurrence of heartburn, dyspepsia, dyspnoea, orthopnoea or hernias (abdominal or inguinal)? Suggests ascites or abdominal masses.
6. Is the swelling painful? Generalised abdominal swelling causes discomfort in the flanks and groins and low back ache; localised pain suggests an enlarged viscus; visceral pain with swelling suggests a bowel disorder.

Investigations

A careful history and examination usually suggests the cause and therefore the appropriate investigations.

ASCITES

This is the accumulation of free fluid in the peritoneal cavity.

Causes of ascites

Transudation

  Hypoalbumininaemia (of any cause) — e.g. nephrotic syndrome, chronic liver disease, burns, malnutrition, GI protein loss.

  High venous pressure

  Systemic, e.g. right heart failure, inferior vena caval obstruction, constrictive pericarditis.

  Portal — *presinusoidal*, e.g. portal vein thrombosis, myelofibrosis
  sinusoidal e.g. most cases of hepatic cirrhosis
  post-sinusoidal, (may also cause exudate) e.g. hepatic vein thrombosis (Budd–Chiari syndrome), veno-occlusive disease.

Exudation

  Inflammatory process (of any cause) — e.g. bacterial peritonitis, pancreatitis, tuberculosis, mesenteric vascular occlusion, starch peritonitis.

Peritoneal malignancy — usually secondary to carcinoma of colon, stomach, ovary, pancreas or any metastatic disease affecting peritoneum or liver.

Myxoedema

Other — such as chylous ascites, pancreatic ascites.

Important questions

1. Is it ascites? Large ovarian cysts may be mistaken for ascites
2. Is the ascites infected? Primary peritonitis is a common complication of ascites especially if caused by chronic liver disease (cirrhosis). Signs of peritonism and even fever are commonly absent or low grade.
3. What is the protein content of the ascites? Protein concentrations <30 g/l suggest a transudate and >30 g/l suggest an exudate.
4. Is the ascites blood stained? Cytology of ascitic fluid can be difficult and misleading. Blood staining is highly suggestive of secondary malignancy or, in cirrhosis, of hepatoma.

Investigations

History and full clinical examination will often suggest the cause. Pay particular attention to any suggestive evidence of:

Heart failure — especially raised JVP

Infection — temperature

Malignancy — weight loss, faecal occult blood test

Chronic liver disease — spider naevi, jaundice, etc.

Portal hypertension — splenomegaly, distended veins

Haematological disease — anaemia, splenomegaly, lymphadenopathy

1. Full blood count including white cell count, blood cultures, serum albumin, liver function tests, amylase, alphafetoprotein.
2. Urinalysis for protein.
3. Diagnostic paracentesis (note colour) to obtain fluid for white cell count, culture, protein concentration, microscopy and cytology, amylase content, special tests — microscopy for starch grains, alpha-fetoprotein for hepatoma, Sudan red stain for fat (chylous ascites).
4. Ultrasonic scan of liver and pancreas for evidence of hepatic or pancreatic malignancy, cirrhosis or to confirm presence of ascites in difficult cases (obesity, ovarian cyst).
5. Laparoscopy (and biopsy) indicated for diagnosis of peritoneal disease and either focal (e.g. malignancy) or diffuse (e.g. cirrhosis) liver disease in the presence of ascites.
6. Isotope liver scan.
   Characteristic appearance in hepatic vein thrombosis.

Useful in locating hepatoma (which is usually 'cold' on technetium scanning).

7. Hepatic venography — indicated in suspected Budd-Chiari syndrome

8. In difficult cases consider cardiac investigations or measurement of GI protein loss.

4. ABDOMINAL PAIN AND THE ACUTE ABDOMEN

ABDOMINAL PAIN

There are numerous causes of abdominal pain. Specific diseases causing abdominal pain are dealt with in the appropriate chapters and only general principles are considered here.

Definition

Pain is a perception which, unlike most senses, is able to intrude rapidly into consciousness. Peripheral pain is commonly experienced in the normal traumas of early life, and the developing child soon learns to associate it with noxious stimuli. Sensations arising within the abdomen, however, are few. The relationship between noxious stimuli and visceral abdominal pain are much less clear cut than with peripheral pain so that the opportunities for the developing human to learn the significance of certain visceral sensations are insubstantial. Consequently, sensations arising from abdominal viscera, which are described as 'pain', do not necessarily have the same ominous significance for the health of the individual as does peripheral pain. Visceral abdominal pain may indicate organic disease, e.g. cholecystitis; but it is common for sensations, which are perceived as pain by the patient, to have no organic cause, e.g. irritable bowel syndrome. Skill and experience in assessing all aspects of a patient's symptoms are therefore of particular importance in determining the significance of abdominal pain. It is equally important to understand that advanced pathology may be present in an abdomen in the total absence of perceived pain.

Causes of abdominal pain

Common gastrointestinal causes
1. Functional (non-organic) pain
2. Inflammatory disease
   non-specific, e.g. appendicitis, diverticulitis
   specific infection, e.g. campylobacter enteritis
   secondary infection, e.g. cholecystitis

idiopathic, e.g. Crohn's disease
autodigestive, e.g. pancreatitis, peptic ulcer
Mechanical or obstructive
    calculus
    acute or chronic inflammation
    stricture
    neoplasm
    volvulus
    extrinsic compression
Ischaemia/infarction
    involving serosal surface, e.g. spleen, small bowel
Emergencies
    perforation
    haemorrhage
    rupture

Malignant abdominal neoplasms
These are rarely a cause of pain unless or until mechanical obstruction develops, ischaemia or inflammation in related organs supervenes or extension occurs beyond the visceral peritoneum when the pain has the features of non-visceral pain.

Pain referred to the abdomen
This may occur secondary to extra-abdominal disease — e.g. myocardial disease (epigastrium), pleural disease (upper abdomen), spinal disease (girdle or root pain situated according to spinal level involved). Metabolic causes include lead poisoning, uraemia, diabetic ketoacidosis and porphyria. Neurogenic causes include herpes zoster and tabes dorsalis.

Important questions

What is the duration and timing of the pain?
1. Sudden recent onset of severe abdominal pain suggests an abdominal emergency e.g. perforation, cholecystitis, appendicitis etc. See 'Acute Abdomen'. Long standing pain in a fit patient suggests functional abdominal pain.
2. Night pain (awakening from sleep) suggests an organic cause.
3. Periodicity of pain in weeks/months is suggestive of certain specific diseases, e.g. peptic ulceration.
4. Cyclical pain is suggestive of gynaecological causes.
5. Episodic, unpredictable attacks are suggestive of biliary tract disease.
6. Pain precipitated by eating is suggestive of upper gastrointestinal disease, e.g. gastric carcinoma, peptic ulcer disease.
7. Pain precipitated by certain specific foods, e.g. fat is not diagnostically helpful.
8. Relief by defaecation is suggestive of colonic pain.

What is the site of the pain?
There is enormous variability between patients in the site at which pain
may be perceived in any single disease — particularly colonic and biliary
tract disease. Some of the more common sites are indicated below:

1. Stomach/duodenum — epigastrium, left hypochondrium and
   back.
2. Pancreas — epigastrium, back and either loin.
3. Gall bladder — right hypochondrium, epigastrium, scapulae,
   shoulder.
4. Small intestine — umbilical region.
5. Colon — epigastrium, hypochondrium, flanks, iliac fossae.
6. Ovaries, uterus, bladder — hypogastrium, left or right iliac
   fossae.
7. Aorta — umbilical region, back, either loin.
8. Kidney, ureter — loin, inguinal region, penis/vulva.
9. Peritoneum — accurately localised to the site of involvement,
   e.g. right iliac fossa in diverticulitis, left iliac fossa in
   appendicitis.

What is the character of the pain?
This can be diagnostically helpful in certain characteristic diseases, e.g.
the gnawing pain of peptic ulceration or the colicky pain of intestinal and
ureteric disease.

Are there any associated symptoms?
These may vary considerably according to the organ involved. Examples
include:

1. Systemic symptoms such as fever — suggests
   inflammation/infection e.g. Crohn's disease, cholecystitis.
2. Weight loss and anaemia — common in gastrointestinal
   malignancy.
3. Diabetes mellitus — complicates pancreatic disease.
4. Jaundice — hepatobiliary disease.

Are there important emotional aspects?
These are common as a primary feature in functional abdominal pain,
but may occur secondary to organic disease.

Diagnosis

There is no other field in medicine in which the diagnosis depends so
heavily on an accurate, detailed and sympathetic history obtained by an
experienced physician. Physical signs may be subtle. Physical examination
must always include digital rectal examination, a test for occult blood on
the faeces, a sigmoidoscopy if appropriate, and clinical examination of the
urine.

   Remember that 50% of patients with abdominal pain have no organic
disease, but the diagnosis of functional abdominal pain is, like the

diagnosis of organic disease, based on the presence of positive diagnostic features (e.g. very long history, multiple abdominal sites, abdominal bloating etc.) and not on the mere absence of objective signs of organic disease.

Investigations

1. Clinical
   a. Temperature
   b. Urinalysis for protein, blood,
      bile etc.
   c. Faecal occult blood test
   d. Sigmoidoscopy
2. Blood
   a. Full blood count, ESR, acute phase proteins
   b. Serum proteins, liver function tests
3. Specific investigations
   See appropriate chapter

Remember, in functional abdominal pain *multiple* investigations yielding normal results:
1. Never 'exclude' organic disease
2. Never 'reassure' the patient
3. Commonly increase the patient's frustration

THE ACUTE ABDOMEN

The acute abdomen is a term applied to the symptoms and signs of abdominal pain and tenderness which are in themselves nonspecific but which are commonly present in a patient presenting with an acute intra-abdominal catastrophe.

Causes of the acute abdomen

Perforation of abdominal viscus
Common perforations include:
   Stomach, due to peptic ulcer or neoplasm
   Duodenum, due to peptic ulcer
   Colon, due to diverticular disease, carcinoma, acute ulcerative colitis, obstruction, necrosis secondary to vascular occlusion
   Appendix, secondary to acute appendicitis
   Gallbladder, due to obstruction and sepsis consequent on cholelithiasis or occasionally malignancy

Small intestine, due to vascular occlusion necrosis, obstruction and occasionally malignancy, e.g. lymphoma.

Acute pancreatitis
Due to:
>Biliary tract disease
>Alcohol abuse
>Secondary to certain drugs (steroids, thiazides, etc.)
>Hypercalcaemia Hypothermia
>Idiopathic causes

Acute cholecystitis
>Usually secondary to cholelithiasis but can be acalculous

Acute appendicitis
>Especially in the younger patient

Intestinal obstruction
>Small intestinal obstruction — due to adhesions from previous surgery, obstructed herniae
>Large intestinal obstruction — due to adhesions from previous surgery, colonic carcinoma, diverticular disease, obstructed herniae, volvulus of sigmoid colon

Intra-abdominal haemorrhage
>Vascular disease — e.g. rupture or dissection of aortic aneurysm
>Disorders of coagulation — e.g. retroperitoneal haemorrhage in poorly controlled therapeutic anticoagulation, haematological diseases associated with thrombocytopaenia, vitamin K deficiency (chronic malabsorption states)
>Traumatic — e.g. rupture of spleen or liver

Metabolic disease Several metabolic diseases can cause a clinical picture indistinguishable from the true acute abdomen, e.g. porphyria, tabetic crises, periodic polyserositis, diabetes mellitus

Differential diagnosis — urinary tract infection, ectopic pregnancy, pelvic inflammatory disease, ureteric colic, shingles, mittelschmerz pain, spinal disease, myocardial infarction, mesenteric adenitis, pneumonia

Important questions

1. Has the patient had previous abdominal surgery?
2. Is there any coexisting disease? Surgical treatment is required for most patients with acute abdominal emergencies. Much of the perioperative mortality is due to pre-existing disease, e.g. cardiac disease, vascular disease, respiratory problems. Their presence influences decisions on suitability for and timing of surgery and influences post-operative management.

Investigations

Careful history and examination including rectal and, where indicated, vaginal examination are mandatory, paying particular attention to abdominal tenderness, guarding, rebound tenderness, masses, bowel sounds and tenderness and the presence of faeces per rectum. Hydration must be assessed and temperature measured.

   Many causes of the acute abdomen (e.g. acute appendicitis, cholecystitis) rely heavily on clinical acumen for diagnosis rather than special investigation

RESUSCITATION OF THE PATIENTS MUST TAKE PRIORITY OVER INVESTIGATIVE PROCEDURES

1. Treat pain with appropriate analgesic.
2. Ensure adequate oxygenation.
3. Correct hypotension by restoring circulating blood volume using whole blood (plasma expanders until available). Correct hydration with crystalloids as necessary.
4. Relieve vomiting by nasogastric aspiration (ileus is an almost universal occurrence in the acute abdomen).

Then:

1. *Blood cultures* — many causes of the acute abdomen are associated with bacteraemia or septicaemia; blood cultures taken early are often useful for later management.
2. *Measure* serum amylase, urea and electrolytes and full blood count; send off MSU and do urinalysis.
3. *Radiology* — plain abdominal erect and supine films. Look for:
   a. Free gas — perforation of viscus.
   b. Dilated bowel with air/fluid levels — intestinal obstruction
      What is the level of the obstruction — large intestinal, small intestinal or generalised (ileus)?
   c. Psoas shadows obscured — possible retroperitoneal pathology.
   d. Calcification in the region of the pancreas (suggesting chronic pancreatitis), biliary tree (suggesting cholelithiasis) or renal tract (suggesting urolithiasis).
4. *Diagnostic paracentesis* — indicated when there is clinical or radiological evidence of free fluid. Aspirate fluid for culture, cytology, protein content and examine aspirate for blood and bile.
5. *Ultrasound scanning*
   Indicated for visualisation in suspected biliary tract disease, pancreatic disease, abdominal and hepatic abscess, detection of free peritoneal fluid.

5. DIARRHOEA, CONSTIPATION AND ANORECTAL SYMPTOMS

DIARRHOEA

This is the passage of loose or watery stools of increased weight, i.e. refers to stool consistency, not to stool frequency. Stricter definitions are more difficult because of the wide variations of normal bowel habit.

Causes of diarrhoea

Infections (acute infective diarrhoea)
>   Viral (commonest) e.g. Rotavirus
>   Bacterial
>   a. Organisms predominantly invasive (mucosal invasion, hence bacteraemia, septicaemia, local or distant abscess formation) e.g. *Campylobacter* species, *Salmonella typhi, Shigella, Yersinia enterocolitica, Neisseria gonorrhoeae.*
>   b. Organisms predominantly toxigenic (mucosal invasive potential limited or insignificant) e.g. *Vibrio cholerae, Clostridium difficile*, some species of *E. coli* and *Salmonella B. Cereus.*
>   Protozoan, *e.g. Giardia lamblia, Entamoeba histiolytica* traveller's diarrhoea.

Inflammatory bowel disease
>   Ulcerative colitis
>   Crohn's disease

Malabsorptive and maldigestive states
>   Pancreatic exocrine failure — pancreatic carcinoma, chronic pancreatitis, fibrocystic disease
>   Hostile luminal environment
>   a. Small bowel bacterial colonisation, e.g. as result of small bowel strictures, entero/gastrocolic fistulae, jejunal diverticula, blind loops, motility disturbance, achlorhydria, partial obstruction, etc.
>   b. Low pH, e.g. Zollinger-Ellison syndrome.

Mucosal disease, e.g. coeliac disease, Crohn's disease, Whipple's disease, tropical sprue, abetalipoproteinaemia, immunodeficiency states, lymphangiectasia, radiation enteritis.

Bile salt deficiency, e.g. intrahepatic or extrahepatic cholestasis, terminal ileal resections, chronic liver diseases, biliary diversions, bile salt destruction (resulting from small bowel bacterial colonisation) bile salt sequestering agents.

Ischaemia, e.g. atheromatous disease, radiation damage, systemic sclerosis, vasculitis.

Specific biochemical deficiency states, e.g. disaccharidase deficiency (alactasia, etc.), amino acid transport deficiencies, congenital chloridorrhoea.

Unknown and multifactorial mechanisms, e.g. systemic sclerosis, diabetes mellitus, thyrotoxicosis.

Motility and psychophysiological disorders
Irritable bowel syndrome (IBS)
Anxiety
Autonomic neuropathy

Drug induced
Iatrogenic, e.g. antacids, antibiotics, nonsteroidal anti-inflammatory drugs, digoxin, adrenergic blocking drugs, cholestyramine
Laxative abuse

Hormonal diarrhoeas
Carcinoid syndrome, thyrotoxicosis, medullary thyroid carcinoma, pancreatic endocrine tumours (Verner–Morrison syndrome, Zollinger–Ellison syndrome, glucagonoma syndromes, etc.)

Tumours of gastrointestinal tract
Colorectal carcinoma, villous adenomata, etc.

Surgery
Gastric resection, vagotomy, intestinal resection and bypass.

Miscellaneous
Ischaemia
Irradiation
Spurious diarrhoea secondary to constipation
Food intolerance

Mechanisms

It is often more helpful, particularly for the more difficult diagnostic problems, to think in terms of mechanisms of diarrhoea rather than specific disease entities. Many diseases cause diarrhoea via several mechanisms. This may make the classification of the diarrhoea more difficult but frequently suggests useful therapeutic manoeuvres.

Osmotic diarrhoea
> Malabsorbed nutrients
> Saline purgatives
> Unabsorbed carbohydrate, e.g. lactulose, sorbitol.

Secretory diarrhoea
> Exogenous secretagogues
> 1. Enterotoxins, e.g. infection with some species of *Salmonellae, Staphylococci, Vibrio cholerae*, etc.
> 2. Dietary derived e.g. free long chain fatty acids and dihydroxy bile acids in malabsorption states.
> Endogenous secretagogues
> 1. Hormonal/peptide diarrhoeas, e.g. carcinoid tumours, gastrinomas, medullary thyroid carcinoma, VIP producing tumours, neuroblastomas.
> 2. Villous adenoma.

Other mechanisms
> Exudation, e.g. inflammatory bowel disease.
> Altered motility, e.g. scleroderma.
> Specific ion malabsorption (very rare).

Important questions

1. Does the patient truly have diarrhoea?
   a. Increased stool frequency and incontinence commonly confused with diarrhoea.
   b. Consider purgative abuse.
   c. Is there spurious diarrhoea?
2. Is the diarrhoea likely to be infective in origin? Does the patient have fever, malaise, rigors, colicky abdominal pain, blood or pus in the stool, vomiting, burning or scalding on passing a motion?
3. Is the diarrhoea likely to be small bowel or large bowel in origin?
   a. Large bowel diarrhoea is often watery, very frequent, small in amounts, produces marked urgency, incontinence or tenesmus or is associated with pain in the flanks and hypogastrium.
   b. Small bowel diarrhoea is often a semi-formed, less frequent, large and bulky stool, often has features of steatorrhoea or is associated with pain in the centre of the abdomen.
4. Is the diarrhoea associated with clinical features of malabsorption?
   a. Steatorrhoeic stool (pale, bulky, greasy, offensive, etc.).
   b. Anaemia (especially mixed deficiency anaemias).
   c. Cutaneous changes (skin rashes, hair loss, nail changes).
   d. Metabolic bone disease (especially osteomalacia).

   e. Clotting deficiency (especially prolonged prothrombin time).

   f. Wasting, weight loss, myopathy.

   g. Oedema.

5. Is the diarrhoea influenced by food intake?

   a. On fasting, stool volume unchanged— secretory diarrhoea very probable.

   b. On fasting, stool volume decreased— osmotic diarrhoea very probable.

6. Is the diarrhoea nocturnal? — This suggests organic rather than functional diarrhoea.

7. Is the diarrhoea related to ingestion of any particular food?

8. Are any of the following symptoms associated — pain, tenesmus, bleeding, abdominal swelling, weight loss, rectal burning, mucus per rectum?

9. Enquire about previous medical history (especially operations and health as child), drug history, foreign travel, contacts (sexual or otherwise) with people with diarrhoea.

Examinations

1. Assessment of hydration and nutritional status.

2. Temperature — fever suggests infection, inflammatory bowel disease, malignancy.

3. Rectal examination.

4. Test for occult blood — positive test indicates breach of mucosal integrity, e.g. infection, inflammatory bowel disease, malignancy.

5. Sigmoidoscopy and biopsy

   a. Ulcerative colitis always visible in rectum.

   b. The majority (55%) of colorectal carcinomas are within reach of the 25 cm sigmoidoscope.

   c. Biopsy of a normal looking mucosa sometimes detects unsuspected disease, e.g., amyloid, Crohn's disease, melanosis coli. *N.B.* Mild reddening of the rectal mucosa is common in anyone with chronic diarrhoea; it does not necessarily indicate proctitis.

The cause of the diarrhoea is often apparent from a full history and examination or, at least, the area of the gastrointestinal tract causing the diarrhoea, may be ascertained.

Investigations

Investigation is necessary in severe acute diarrhoea and in all chronic diarrhoeas (i.e. diarrhoea persisting for more than two weeks).

1. *Examine the stool*

   a. Is it diarrhoea?

    b. Is there macroscopic or microscopic pus or blood? —
      infection, inflammatory bowel disease, diverticulitis, etc. Is
      there altered food or mucus?

    c. Stool culture for pathogens including *Campylobacter,*
      Clostridium difficile, Yersinia.

    d. Microscopy for pus cells, parasites, protozoa, fat globules.

2. *Routine blood tests*
   Full blood count, differential white cell count, blood film, acute
   phase proteins, ESR, blood urea and electrolytes, serum liver
   function tests, calcium, magnesium, proteins, iron, B_{12}, and red cell
   folate.

3. *Radiology*
    a. Barium enema — if history and physical examination suggest
      colonic disease and there is no colitis on sigmoidoscopy

    b. Barium follow through (not meal!) — if history suggests
      small bowel disease, or if malabsorption appears to be
      present.

4. *Fibreoptic colonoscopy* — used
    a. To clarify suspicious areas on radiology.

    b. Assess mucosal disease and obtain biopsy.

    c. Assess colon in radiologically negative diarrhoea.

5. *If malabsorption, maldigestion or steatorrhoea is suspected*:
    (*N.B.*. a normal looking stool does not exclude steatorrhoea!)

    a. Is malabsorption present? — measure faecal fat output on
      100 g fat diet. Faecal fat > 15 mmol stearic acid/day indicates
      malabsorption (steatorrhoea). Remember to complete faecal
      fat collection before doing barium studes; barium interferes
      with the measurement of faecal fat.

    b. What is the disease causing the malabsorption?
      First perform barium follow through.
      If normal then — perform jejunal biopsy.
      If normal then — consider performing function tests of small
      intestine.
      Next perform anatomical and functional test of pancreas.
      If normal — assess hepatobiliary (?cholestasis) or gastric
      (?Zollinger–Ellison syndrome) structure and function.

6. *For persistent diarrhoea and negative investigation:*
    a. Admit to hospital (if not already there), correct fluid and
      electrolyte deficits and measure daily stool outputs.

    b. Fast the patient and measure daily stool output again
      (maintain hydration with i.v. fluids).

      (i) If the daily stool volume decreases on fasting — suggests
         malabsorption, hostile luminal environment, bile salt
         deficiency states, etc.

      (ii) If there is no change in stool volume on fasting —
         suggests a secretory diarrhoea.

   Then measure the electrolyte content of stool water and

calculate expected osmolality (sodium plus potassium concentration ×2 to allow for anions) and then measure the actual osmolality of the stool water.

If the *calculated* osmolality *equals observed* osmolality, look for causes of secretory diarrhoea (pancreatic VIP tumour, enterotoxin producing organisms, thyroid carcinoma, etc.)

If *observed* osmolality significantly *exceeds calculated* osmolality, look for causes of osmotic diarrhoea (concealed purgative abuse, malabsorption, etc.)

c. Further special tests may be needed in difficult cases, e.g. arteriography, CT scanning, intestinal perfusion, laparotomy, therapeutic trials.

CONSTIPATION

It is vital to define exactly what the patient means by constipation. Normal bowel habits are very variable but defaecation less than three times a week is probably always abnormal. However, passage of rock like stools and the need to strain at stool also indicate constipation, even if the patient defaecates relatively frequently. Of most importance is the change from a previously well established bowel habit. Remember that patients may complain of constipation when they mean tenesmus. Women more often complain of constipation than men.

Causes of constipation

Colorectal disease
> Simple rectal constipation (habitual failure to answer urge to defaecate; also called psychogenic constipation)
> Slow transit constipation (colonic inertia without megacolon)
> Irritable bowel syndrome
> Diverticular disease
> Hirschsprung's disease (classical, short segment or ultra-short segment)
> Other causes of aganglionosis e.g. Chagas' disease, pseudo–obstruction
> Colonic malignancy
> Intestinal obstruction
> Painful anal and perianal lesions

Proximal gastrointestinal disease
> Gastric carcinoma
> Coeliac disease

Weakness or damage to perineal muscles
> Systemic illness
> Ageing

Neurological disease
Pelvic or spinal trauma

Neurological disease
Parkinson's disease
Cerebrovascular disease
Multiple sclerosis
Autonomic neuropathy

Metabolic disease
Diabetes mellitus
Uraemia
Dehydration
Hypokalaemia
Hypothyroidism
Hypercalcaemia
Porphyria

Drugs
e.g. opiates, aluminium salts, barium salts, anticholingergics, iron, methotrexate

Toxins
e.g. lead

Psychiatric disease
Depression
Anorexia nervosa

Fever

Pregnancy

N.B. Megacolon is not a cause of constipation but rather a result of certain causes of constipation, e.g. Hirschsprung's disease, other causes of aganglionosis, life long simple constipation.

Important questions

1. How severe is the constipation? Assessed by stool frequency, need to strain, passage of 'rocks' and the need for digital evacuation.
2. Is the constipation of recent onset or is it long standing? A history from the mother is helpful in evaluating long standing constipation in a child or young adult. Lifelong constipation suggests the possiblity of Hirschsprung's disease, slow transit constipation or simple rectal constipation (with or without megacolon). Remember Hirschsprung's disease (especially the short segment type) may not appear until later childhood or adult life.
3. Is the constipation complete? Suggests intestinal obstruction.
4. Is the constipation associated with pain? Abdominal pain suggests obstruction, carcinoma, IBS, diverticular disease or porphyria; perianal pain suggests a local anal disorder.

5. Is the constipation associated with vomiting? Suggests intestinal obstruction, hypercalcaemia or uraemia.
6. Does the constipation alternate with loose stools? Suggests colonic carcinoma, IBS, diverticular disease or faecal impaction with overflow ('spurious' diarrhoea). Remember constipation may present with 'spurious' diarrhoea.
7. Is the patient taking any drugs?
8. Is there any neurological or spinal disease or any history of injury to the pelvis or lower spine?

Investigations

1. Physical examination must include:
   Perineal inspection — looking for painful lesions etc.
   Rectal examination — noting anal tone, squeeze pressure and whether rectum is empty or capacious and full of faeces.
2. Sigmoidoscopy — looking for local lesions (e.g. carcinoma) and evidence of melanosis coli.
3. Faecal occult blood.
4. Full blood count, ESR.
5. Blood urea, electrolytes, calcium, thyroid function tests.
6. Radiology
   a. Plain abdominal X-ray — necessary in suspected obstruction; will show faecal loading.
   b. Barium enema — indicated in all cases unless severe obstruction is present or the cause is obvious; may reveal causative lesion, megacolon, or typical appearance of Hirschsprung's disease.
7. Special investigation — indicated in difficult cases especially where there is a long history.
   a. Rectal biopsy — should be deep enough to demonstrate whether the myenteric plexus ganglion cells are present, absent or damaged.
   b. Anorectal and colonic manometry and colonic transit studies — indicated in long standing constipation without obvious cause and with or without megacolon.

ANORECTAL SYMPTOMS

Tenesmus
This is the uncomfortable sensation of incomplete evacuation of the rectum after defaecation. It is sometimes called rectal dissatisfaction. It is *not* painful defaecation.

Causes

Rectal inflammation of any cause
Constipation

Rectal tumours
Irritable bowel syndrome

Rectal bleeding

Bright red blood per rectum suggests anorectal bleeding but brisk bleeding from higher in the GI tract may cause fresh blood per rectum. Anal canal bleeding usually follows defaecation or blood covers the stool and is not mixed with it. Passage of blood without stool may be a feature of rectal bleeding.

Causes

Haemorrhoids
Anorectal tumours
Proctitis and/or distal colitis
Solitary ulcer of the rectum
Fissure–in–ano
Trauma, e.g. sexual, digital, etc.

Anal pain

Causes

Fissure–in–ano
Perianal haematoma
Perianal abscess
Haemorrhoids
Irritable bowel syndrome
Proctalgia fugax
Anorectal tumours

Local anal lesions tend to cause pain at defaecation whereas IBS and proctalgia cause pain at other times and proctalgia fugax causes pain typically during the night.

Pruritus ani

In 50% of patients, no cause is identifiable but possible aetiological factors are obesity, chemicals in food, psychogenic disorders.

Causes which are identifiable

Anorectal discharge of any cause
Frequent stools
Infection, e.g. threadworms, candida
Skin disease, e.g. psoriasis
Drugs, e.g. colchicine

Faecal incontinence

Causes

Faecal impaction in elderly or ill
Anorectal disease, e.g. prolapse
haemorrhoids
tumours
Crohn's disease

Neurological disease
Psychiatric disease
Trauma (accidental, operative or obstetric) to anal ring and
   sphincters
Severe watery diarrhoea of any cause
Congenital

Soiling
This results from discharge from the anus or perianal area onto
underwear.

Causes

Any of the causes of incontinence
Discharge from fistulae or sinuses, e.g. Crohn's disease
Drugs especially liquid paraffin

N.B. Anorectal symptoms, especially incontinence and soiling, are often
embarrassing to the patient who does not volunteer them. Therefore
direct enquiry is necessary.

Investigation of anorectal symptoms

1. Careful inspection of anus and perineum.
2. Rectal examination and faecal occult blood test.
3. Proctoscopy.
4. Sigmoidoscopy and, if appropriate, rectal biopsy.
5. Swab discharges and pus or mucus on anorectal mucosa.
6. Stool microscopy and culture.
7. Special tests, e.g. anal manometry in special circumstances.

6. JAUNDICE

Jaundice is a yellow colouration of skin and mucous membranes caused by an abnormal increase in the serum bilirubin level. Jaundice is not usually visible until the serum bilirubin is greater than 45 μmol/l.

Causes

Bilirubin is produced in the reticuloendothelial system from haemoglobin released by effete red cells. It is unconjugated and therefore insoluble in water. It is bound to albumin and transported to the liver where it is taken up into the liver cell, conjugated with glucuronic acid and then excreted into bile in the biliary canaliculi. These drain ultimately into the duodenum via the hepatic and common bile ducts. Jaundice may therefore be:

1. *Prehepatic*
   This may be due to increased rate of bilirubin production in excess of the hepatic uptake, as in haemolysis, or impaired hepatic uptake of bilirubin, e.g. Gilbert's syndrome.
2. *Posthepatic*
   Obstruction to the biliary flow ('cholestasis'). The obstruction may be extrahepatic, i.e. distal to the porta hepatis, or intrahepatic, i.e. proximal to the porta hepatis.
3. *Hepatic*
   Caused by damage to the liver cell, acute or chronic.

N.B. Many common causes of jaundice are of mixed aetiology, e.g. drugs, sepsis.

Important questions

1. Has the patient been jaundiced before?
2. Has the patient had any blood transfusions or injections in the last six months?
3. Has the patient been abroad or had any contacts (sexual or otherwise) with a jaundiced patient? Is the patient homosexual?
4. What drugs has the patient been taking? Is there a history of drug abuse? What is the alcohol consumption?

5. Is the patient a cross infection risk?
Examine blood for HBsAg and HBe Ag
6. Is the jaundice prehepatic?
Urine normal in colour.
Negative test for bilirubin in urine.
Liver function tests normal other than bilirubin level.
Confirm by measuring serum conjugated and unconjugated
bilirubin level ('direct and indirect' bilirubin).
Consider:
 a. Haemolysis — haemoglobin level, MCV, reticulocyte
    count, methaemalbumin, etc.
 b. Gilbert's syndrome and its variants (common) — confirm
    with nicotinic acid provocation if necessary.
7. Is the jaundice cholestatic?
Urine dark in colour.
Positive test for bilirubin in urine.
Faeces may be pale depending on degree of cholestasis.
Pruritus common.
Pain — often in extrahepatic obstruction.
If there are features of cholestasis, then consider:
 a. At what level is the cholestasis occurring?
    Extrahepatic cholestasis (bile duct strictures,
       choledocholithiasis, neoplasms of ampulla and pancreas,
       etc.) commonly necessitates surgical intervention.
    Intrahepatic cholestasis commonly affects the small biliary
       canaliculi and is rarely amenable to surgery.
 b. Is there any evidence of co-existing sepsis?
    Fever
    Leucocytosis
    Blood cultures
    N.B Sepsis in the presence of biliary obstruction
    — Is an emergency carrying a high mortality, requires
       urgent and rapid treatment with antibiotics and possibly
       surgery. Diabetics are at considerably increased risk.
    — Makes investigation (e.g. endoscopic cholangiography)
       dangerous.
8. Is the jaundice hepatic in origin?
 a. Mixed features often with a major cholestatic component.
 b. Clinical and biochemical evidence of liver disease which
    may be:
    i. Acute, e.g. viral or drug induced hepatitis.
    ii. Chronic, e.g. cirrhosis of any cause.
If a hepatic cause for jaundice seems likely, then consider:
    Is hepatic failure present (fluid retention, encephalopathy,
       bleeding from clotting deficiency)?
    Is any complication present, e.g. portal hypertension?

Investigations

Physical examination must include

1. Temperature — infection in the biliary tree must not be missed
2. Search for relevant signs:
   a. Pigmentation — suggests longstanding cholestatic jaundice.
   b. Leuconychia, spider naevi, palmar erythema, gynaecomastia, testicular atrophy, etc. suggesting chronic liver disease.
   c. Easy bruising, oedema, confusion, flapping tremor, etc., suggesting liver failure.
   d. Splenomegaly, ascites, suggesting portal hypertension
   e. Injection marks, home made tattoos, evidence of alcohol abuse (such as topers facies, etc.), scratch marks.
3. Examination of urine for bilirubin and excessive urobilinogen and faeces for colour and presence of occult blood.

Haematological examination

1. Full blood count including differential WCC; coagulation screen (platelet count, prothrombin time, activated partial thromboplastin time).
2. HBsAg and HBeAg to eliminate cross infection risk early.
3. Liver function tests:
   a. Serum bilirubin — conjugated or unconjugated; if unconjugated exclude haemolysis.
   b. Alkaline phosphatase — disproportionately raised in cholestasis (both intrahepatic and extrahepatic) and space occupying lesions, e.g. metastatic liver disease, hepatic abscess.
   c. Aspartate amino-transferase — high levels indicate hepatocellular damage of any cause. Very high levels suggest a diffuse hepatitis (e.g. viral or drug damage). Moderate elevations in severe or longstanding cholestasis. Mild elevation in established, nonactive cirrhosis.
   d. Serum albumin — decreased in extensive liver impairment either acute or chronic.
   e. Serum globulin — moderate increase in the presence of low albumin suggests chronic liver disease such as cirrhosis. Marked elevations suggest chronic active liver disease.
4. Autoantibodies — nonspecific markers occurring transiently and in low titre in many situations of liver damage. Persistent high titres suggest 'autoimmune' liver disease, e.g. antinuclear antibody and smooth muscle antibody in chronic active hepatitis, antimitochondrial antibody in primary biliary cirrhosis.

5. Prothrombin time — can be prolonged in any cause of jaundice other than prehepatic. Important to correct before invasive investigations. Phytomenadione parenterally rapidly corrects prolongations caused by cholestatic disease.
6. Alphafetoprotein — high titre suggests hepatoma.

Hepatic ultrasound examination

Particularly useful and particularly indicated in the presence of cholestasis.

1. No dilatation of intrahepatic bile ducts — suggests intrahepatic cholestasis. Proceed to percutaneous liver biopsy once coagulation parameters have been restored to normal.
2. Dilatation of intra or extrahepatic biliary tree visible — suggests extrahepatic cholestasis. Then ensure that coagulation has been restored, take blood cultures and start prophylactic antibiotics in preparation for either endoscopic retrograde cholangiopancreatography (ERCP) or percutaneous transhepatic cholangiography (PTC) using Chiba needle to visualise biliary tree.
3. Scan suggests focal liver disease, e.g. hepatic metastases. Then:
   a. Ensure coagulation is restored.
   b. Perform percutaneous liver biopsy.

Liver biopsy

Indicated after correction of coagulation deficiencies for:

1. Accurate diagnosis of hepatitis — drug induced, viral, etc.
2. Accurate diagnosis of intrahepatic cholestasis — benign intrahepatic, drug induced, primary biliary cirrhosis, etc.
3. Accurate diagnosis of focal liver disease under ultrasonic or laparoscopic control — hepatoma, metastatic liver disease.

Bromsulphthalein retention test

Of little value except in the uncommon congenital conjugated hyperbilirubinaemias (Dubin–Johnson syndrome and its variants) when reexcretion of the dye into the serum by the liver in the prolonged test is diagnostic.

PART TWO
Diagnosis and Treatment

7. OESOPHAGEAL DISEASE

GASTRO OESOPHAGEAL REFLUX

This is related to a number of factors but the main ones are probably lowering of the lower oesophageal sphincter (LOS) pressure and impairment of secondary oesophageal peristalsis which clears refluxed material from the oesophagus. All individuals reflux asymptomatically to a mild degree at some time but symptoms result from failure of these two mechanisms which lead to prolonged and frequent episodes of reflux. Reflux of gastric contents causes reflux oesophagitis. The damage is caused by acid and pepsin and in some individuals by bile refluxed into the stomach from the duodenum. The presence or absence of a sliding hiatal hernia is much less important in reflux than was once thought; a majority of patients who reflux have no demonstrable hiatal hernia and many patients with radiological hiatal hernias do not complain of reflux symptoms.

Symptoms — Heartburn, regurgitation, dyspepsia, oesophageal pain, and symptoms of gastrointestinal blood loss and pulmonary aspiration. Dysphagia usually only appears with stricture formation.

Signs — Nil

Diagnosis — Reflux is usually strongly suggested by the history. Investigations provide objective evidence of reflux in most cases.

Investigations

Reflux is assessed from four aspects:
  1. Is there reflux?
     Barium swallow
     Radio isotope scan
     pH probe studies and manometry
  2. Is the reflux causing damage?
     Oesophagoscopy and biopsy
  3. Are the symptoms due to reflux?
     Bernstein test — rarely required except in the occasional patient with atypical symptoms.

4. Is a hiatal hernia present?
   Barium swallow and meal — knowledge of the presence of a hiatal hernia is really only required is surgery is to be considered.

There is a poor correlation between symptoms, evidence of reflux, oesophageal damage and the presence of a hiatal hernia.

Treatment

General Measures

Stop smoking
Avoid alcohol
Avoid high fat meals
Avoid food two hours before retiring
Avoid big meals
Prop head of bed up 15–30 cm (6–12 inches)
Lose weight — if appropriate

Specific Measures

1. Increasing LOS pressure — Metoclopramide or cholinergics (e.g. bethanicol) raise LOS pressure but are disappointing in clinical trials. Alkalinization of gastric contents raises LOS pressure but requires large doses of liquid antacid.
2. Modification of refluxed material — H_2 receptor antagonists reduce gastric acid and effectively relieve symptoms in many patients. Large doses of liquid antacid (e.g. Al/Mg mixtures) effectively reduce gastric acid but are less well tolerated. H_2 receptor antagonists also decrease pepsin production. Binding of intragastric bile salts with cholestyramine or aluminium hydroxide gel has not proved very successful in the relief of symptoms.
3. Prevention of reflux. Alginate/antacid mixtures (e.g. Gaviscon, Gastrocote) which may form a film on the gastric juice reducing or preventing reflux often provide great symptomatic relief.
4. Increasing mucosal resistance — Polymethylsiloxane, which is usually combined with antacid (e.g. Asilone, Polycrol), seems to coat the inflamed oesophageal mucosa and frequently relieves symptoms. Carbenoxolone may enhance oesophageal mucosal resistance by undefined mechanisms, and combined with an antacid, as in Pyrogastrone, does provide relief and heal oesophagitis in some patients. Problems may occur with carbenoxolone side effects, such as salt and water retention and hypokalaemia.

Suggested treatment

1. General measures.
2. Gaviscon 10 ml after meals and before retiring to bed.

3. Cimetidine 400 mg qds, if no improvement after (1) and (2).
4. If no improvement after (1), (2) and (3), try polymethylsiloxane/antacid mixture (but not with alginate mixture, as the polymethylsiloxane will disrupt the alginate film on the surface of the gastric residue) or metoclopramide 10 mg tds or, if there is oesophagitis, Pyrogastrone 1 tablet tds after meals and two tablets at bedtime.

Prognosis

In the majority of patients, it is very good. Improvement occurs in most patients whatever treatment is offered. A small proportion will have continued or recurring symptoms requiring further treatment and a few will require consideration of surgery for intractable symptoms or complications.

Surgery

Indications
Complications (see below) and intractable symptoms — but beware of the patient who has severe symptoms but no objective signs of reflux and the patient with demonstrable reflux who has never been able to cooperate with treatment, e.g. by losing weight. Remember that there is increasing evidence that reflux returns in the years after apparently successful antireflux operations.

Type of operation
There are many different procedures with advantages and disadvantages but the important decision for the physician is to select a surgeon who performs many antireflux operations successfully, rather than select a surgeon because of the particular procedure he does.

Complications

1. *Strictures* — usually present with dysphagia, and are diagnosed by barium swallow and endoscopy with cytology and biopsy. Treatment is often surgical if the patient is fit, or by regular endoscopic dilatation if the patient refuses surgery or is too frail for surgery. With mild strictures, the patient might be happy to continue on a liquidized diet.
2. *Barrett's oesophagus* — consists of columnar mucosa appearing in the distal oesophagus. It is now thought to be a complication of reflux and have malignant potential (possibly about 10% in 10 years). It is diagnosed by endoscopy and biopsy and treated by regular follow up with biopsy and by surgery if histology is suspicious or if there is severe reflux.
3. *Oesophageal ulcer* — a rare complication of reflux which causes severe unremitting epigastric or retrosternal pain

There is a risk of perfortion or bleeding and of healing with stricture formation. Diagnosed by barium swallow and endoscopy with cytology and biopsy. It is treated with general anti–reflux measures, antacids and H_2-receptor antagonists. Surgery is indicated for failure to heal, bleeding, perforation or stricture formation.

4. *Gastrointestinal bleeding* — may present acutely as haematemesis or melaena or as chronic iron deficiency, especially in the elderly. Bleeding comes from oesophagitis, or, more rarely, ulceration. Diagnosis is by endoscopy, full blood count, serum iron, faecal occult bloods and exclusion of other causes of GI bleeding. Treatment consists of replacing blood and iron losses, medical antireflux measures and, occasionally, surgery.

5. *Pulmonary aspiration* — symptoms are coughing, dyspnoea and wheezing, (especially at night) and recurrent attacks of bronchitis or pneumonia. Assessment is by chest X-ray and demonstration of reflux. Prevention of reflux by surgery is probably the treatment of choice.

ACHALASIA

There are two abnormalities, the lower oesophageal sphincter (LOS) fails to relax when food or liquid is swallowed and there is failure of normal peristalsis in the lower two thirds of the oesophagus. The smooth muscle contracts aimlessly or in response to a cholinergic stimulus, but these contractions are non-progressive. Pathologically the circular muscle of the LOS is thickened and there are decreased numbers of ganglion cells in Auerbach's plexuses. The disease can occur at any age but most commonly presents between 20 and 40 years. Histories may go back many years. A positive family history may be obtained.

Symptoms — Dysphagia, regurgitation, aspiration symptoms. Oesophageal colic and odynophagia may occur early in the condition.

Signs — Nil

Complications — Squamous cell carcinoma of the oesophagus (2–7% of large series).

Diagnosis — Typical appearance is seen on barium swallow; endoscopy, biopsy and cytology excludes a malignant or benign stricture. Marked oesophageal contraction in response to methacholine may be shown fluoroscopically or on manometric studies.

Treatment — Heller's myotomy or pneumatic bag dilatation — both can lead to troublesome gastro-oesophageal reflux and dilatation can cause oesophageal rupture. Better long term results with myotomy. Emptying the oesophagus by means of lowering the LOS pressure with nitrates is not a satisfactory treatment.

DIFFUSE SPASM

This may be a variant of achalasia. It is relatively uncommon and is usually seen in elderly patients.

Symptoms — Severe oesophageal colic, which may be precipitated by swallowing or by lying down, and is severe enough to mimic cardiac pain; and dysphagia which may be severe enough to lead to severe weight loss.

Diagnosis — Typical 'corkscrew' appearance of lower two thirds of the oesophagus is seen on barium swallow (*Note* — same appearance may be seen in asymptomatic patients). Prolonged uncoordinated 'tertiary' contractions can be demonstrated manometrically and in most patients may be precipitated by methacholine.

Treatment — Unsatisfactory. Nitrites or nifedipine may help some patients; pneumatic dilatation or, in extreme cases, a long myotomy may be necessary.

OESOPHAGEAL CARCINOMA

95% squamous carcinomas
 5% true adenocarcinomas
Deaths approximately 2 500 per year (England and Wales)
75% of cases — male
70% aged greater than 60 years.

Squamous cell carcinoma

Risk factors may include hot drinks, radiation, achalasia, reflux, alcohol and smoking. There are great racial and geographical differences. There is an association with achalasia, coeliac disease, Patterson–Kelly (Plummer–Vinson) syndrome and tylosis palmaris.
Site — 50% middle third, 25% lower third.

Symptoms
Progressive dysphagia, often with regurgitation, anorexia, malaise, weight loss, blood loss, hoarseness, aspiration symptoms due to overflow or tracheo-oesophageal fistula.

Signs
Early — nil; Late — wasting, hepatomegaly, lymphadenopathy.

Metastases
Commonly to lymph nodes, liver, lung

Complications
Aspiration pneumonia, tracheo-oesophageal fistula, hypercalcaemia, ACTH or gonadotrophin production.

Diagnosis
Barium swallow; endoscopy with biopsy and brush cytology — positive in 96% of cases.

Treatment

1. *Surgery*
   Curative resection — 14–23% 5 year survival, difficult in upper or middle third tumours; Palliative resection — high mortality.
2. *Radiotherapy*
   All patients — 3–10% 5 year survival; highly selected patients — 20% 5 year survival (better for upper or middle third tumours).
3. *Chemotherapy*
   Role in therapy not established
4. *Palliation*
   Palliation is possible by passage of prosthetic tube through tumour — lower mortality with endoscopic insertion than operative insertion. Risks of perforation of oesophagus by prosthesis during insertion and movement of tube occurring after satisfactory placement.

Adenocarcinoma

True oesophageal adenocarcinomas are derived from Barrett's epithelium or oesophageal mucous glands. Most apparent oesophageal adenocarcinomas are in fact fundal gastric carcinomas. Virtually all are found in the distal oesophagus.

Symptoms and Signs
These are similar to squamous carcinoma, although a history of gastro-oesophageal reflux is common.

Treatment
Only chance of prolonged survival is radical total gastrectomy — 22% 5 year survival in highly selected cases but is high operative mortality. The tumour is not radiosensitive; similar palliation as in squamous carcinoma.

8. GASTRODUODENAL DISEASE

PEPTIC ULCER

The maxim 'no acid — no ulcer' still holds true, as does the view that peptic ulcers arise because of a disturbance of the balance between acid output and mucosal resistance. Little else is known. Duodenal ulcer patients tend to have higher than normal acid outputs, whereas gastric ulcer patients tend to have lower than normal outputs. DU is common in males, has a peak prevalence between 45–54 and is getting less common. Remember that duodenal ulcers are quite common in the elderly. They may be associated with chronic renal failure, chronic obstructive airways disease, ischaemic heart disease and hyperparathyroidism. GU is more common in the elderly and is seen equally in both sexes. GU and DU may occur together and prepyloric GU should be considered as a DU from the point of view of treatment.

Symptoms — Epigastric pain and dyspepsia are most common. Nocturnal pain is typical of DU. GU patients tend to lose weight because they may be afraid to eat. DU patients may put on weight because they eat to ease the pain. Vomiting, anorexia, GI bleeding occur. Peptic ulcers may present with their complications, e.g. perforation, acute haemorrhage.

Signs — Epigastric tenderness.

Diagnosis — Demonstration of ulcer by upper GI endoscopy or barium meal (if upper endoscopy is not available).

Investigations

1. Full blood count.
2. Faecal occult blood test.
3. Upper GI endoscopy — gastric, prepyloric and huge duodenal ulcers must be brushed for cytology and biopsied.
4. Special studies — plasma gastrin, serum calcium and acid studies are necessary if ulcer fails to heal, recurs after surgery or if multiple ulcers are present.

Treatment

General measures

Stop smoking as this delays healing. Avoid gastric irritant drugs, e.g. aspirin. No special diets are needed except during an acute severe exacerbation when a light diet with frequent antacid and bed rest as well as specific treatment are necessary.

Specific treatment

Remember 40–50% of peptic ulcers can heal with placebo therapy.

1. *Duodenal ulcer* — the following drugs heal 80% or more of ulcers in 4–6 weeks.
   a. Drugs inhibiting gastric acid output:
   H_2 receptor blockers, e.g. cimetidine, ranitidine
   Pirenzepine
   Trimipramine
   PGE2 analogues
   Omeprazole
   b. Drugs neutralizing gastric acid:
   Aluminium magnesium liquid antacids in large dose (> 200 ml/day)
   c. Drugs promoting mucosal resistance:
   Sucralfate
   Carbenoxolone (as Duogastrone)
   Tripotassium dicitratobismuthate (DeNol)

   The drugs with the lowest incidence of side effects and which have been most widely studied are the H_2 receptor antagonists. There is little to choose between cimetidine (either 400 mg bd or 200 mg tds and 400 mg nocte) or ranitidine (150 mg bd). Ranitidine may have theoretical advantages in the elderly, patients with liver failure and for parenteral use. If these drugs are not well tolerated or fail to heal the DU, a mucosal resistance promoter, e.g. sucralfate (1 g qds) is indicated. DeNol, one tablet tds before meals and two tablets nocte for 28 days has a lower relapse rate than H_2 receptor antagonists.

2. *Gastric ulcer* — the same drugs will heal 60–70% of gastric ulcers over 4–6 weeks. Drugs of choice are the H_2 receptor antagonists with sucralfate as the second choice.

3. *Prepyloric gastric ulcer* — treat as DU.

4. *Pyloric channel ulcer* — treat as DU.

Assessment of ulcer healing

This must be done endoscopically; relief of symptoms does not mean that the ulcer has healed. Always rebiopsy healing or recently healed gastric ulcers as ulcerating gastric carcinomas may temporarily heal on treatment.

Treatment failures

Consider doubling dose of H_2 receptor antagonist, changing to mucosal resistance promoter (e.g. sucralfate) or surgery, which should be particularly considered in patients with non-healing gastric ulcers and in the elderly with any type of non-healing ulcer.

Relapse after healing

Up to 50% of duodenal ulcers relapse in the first year after healing; gastric ulcers also have a high relapse rate. Relapse may be slower after healing with a mucosal resistance promotor than with an H_2 receptor antagonist. Factors associated with relapse are smoking, a long history of peptic ulcer symptoms and a high acid output. Relapse should always suggest the possibility of hypercalcaemia or Zollinger–Ellison Syndrome. After relapse, the ulcer is healed with a further course of a specified treatment. The role of maintenance therapy in preventing relapse has not yet been established. Cimetidine (400 mg nocte) or ranitidine (150 mg nocte) may reduce relapse rates but how long therapy should be given is not known. In older or infirm patients perhaps maintenance should be given for life whereas in younger patients, relapse after a second healing course of treatment should lead to surgery.

Surgery

Types of ulcer healing operation are many and various. The operations of choice are probably: for DU, highly selective vagotomy; and for GU, Billroth I partial gastrectomy.

Complications of peptic ulcer

Haemorrhage

This can be overt, with haematemesis and/or melaena, or occult, leading to iron deficiency anaemia. GI haemorrhage is discussed later.

'Pyloric' stenosis (gastric outflow obstruction)

This may result from a peptic ulcer in the prepyloric area, at the pyloric channel or in the duodenal cap. Other causes are carcinoma, adhesions and hypertrophic pyloric stenosis.

Symptoms

Vomiting without bile but vomit contains food eaten many hours or even days previously; epigastric fullness, discomfort or pain.

Signs

Succussion splash, epigastric tenderness, visible peristalsis, dehydration.

Diagnosis

Diagnosis is suggested by the history and the presence of food in the stomach more than four hours after the last meal; diagnosis is confirmed by a gastric residue of greater than 200 ml after an overnight fast.

Investigations

1. *Barium meal* — barium in the stomach after more than four hours shows delayed gastric emptying; the underlying cause of gastric outflow obstruction may be apparent but often is not.

2. *Upper GI endoscopy* — aspirate stomach first; not always

necessary as most cases go to surgery but may diagnose a carcinoma.

3. *Gastric emptying studies* — rarely indicated in mechanical obstruction to gastric emptying.

4. *Blood urea, electrolytes, acid–base studies and haematocrit* — raised blood urea and haematocrit occur with dehydration; sodium, chloride and potassium may be depressed and a metabolic alkalosis (because of H^+ loss) may be present.

Treatment

1. *Nasogastric suction* — aspirate stomach with wide bore tube and gastric lavage with 200 ml isotonic saline until all food debris is removed; then pass fine nasogastric tube for aspiration 2–4 hourly.

2. *Intravenous fluid and electrolytes*

3. *Surgery* — usually is necessary

4. *Medical* — if pyloric stenosis is due to oedema secondary to an ulcer and the patient is unfit for or unwilling to have surgery, H_2 receptor antagonist therapy can be started and its effectiveness monitored by reduction in the volume of gastric aspirate.

Perforation

Symptoms

Acute severe generalised abdominal pain in a patient who may or may not have a dyspeptic history. Occasionally symptoms of perforation may be minimal, e.g. in elderly or in patients on corticosteroid therapy.

Signs

Scaphoid abdomen with the signs of peritonitis.

Diagnosis

Plain abdominal X–ray (erect) showing free gas under the diaphragm (present in only about 60% patients). In infirm patients, a lateral decubitus film may be possible showing free gas under upper flank.

Treatment

Surgery after any resuscitation that is necessary.

Penetration

Ulcers which break the stomach or duodenal wall but do not perforate are described as penetrating ulcers. Frequently penetration can only be diagnosed at operation. However a penetrating ulcer tends to cause severe intractible epigastric pain which loses periodicity and can cause bleeding. Posterior antral gastric ulcers and posterior duodenal ulcers can penetrate the pancreas causing pancreatic pain and hyperamylasaemia which can be difficult to differentiate from acute pancreatitis.

Treatment

Same as other peptic ulcers; severity of symptoms and occurrence of bleeding often lead to earlier surgery. If pancreatic penetration with hyperamylasaemia is present, treatment as for acute pancreatitis is indicated (see Ch. 11).

GASTRITIS

Acute

There are many causes including:

        Gastric irritants e.g. aspirin, bile
        Systemic illness
        Shock
        Irradiation
        Stress
        Intramucosal bacterial infection (phlegmonous gastritis)

Symptoms
Often present with GI bleed; nausea, epigastric pain and vomiting are less common.

Investigations and diagnosis
Upper GI endoscopy with biopsy (if safe); hyperaemia, acute inflammation and erosions may be seen.

Treatment
Conservative with bed rest, light diet, antacids, H_2 receptor antagonist. Treat and alleviate cause, if possible.

Chronic

This is a confusing topic. Clinically there are probably two groups of patients with gastritis:

1. Patients with parietal cell antibodies, marked impairment of acid secretion leading to B_{12} malabsorption and elevation of plasma gastrin. The antrum is often spared and the gastritis tends to be diffuse. Aetiological factors may be immunological.

2. Patients without parietal cell antibodies, with mild impairment of acid secretion and who have normal plasma gastrin levels, and who rarely develop B_{12} malabsorpiton. The distal stomach is involved and inflammation may be focal. Aetiological factors may include drugs (e.g. alcohol, aspirin), bile, cigarette smoking. This type of gastritis may be associated with peptic ulcer.

Histology
1. Superficial
2. Atrophic — in some patients with pernicious anaemia there is no gastritis and gastric atrophy is a better term.

Both histological types may be seen in either group of patients with gastritis. Metaplasia (intestinal or pseudo pyloric) may be seen with atrophic gastritis in any patient.

Symptoms

The majority of patients are asymptomatic; dyspepsia, epigastric pain or anorexia may occur, especially in Group (2) patients.

Investigations and diagnosis

Upper GI endoscopy with biopsy is the basis of diagnosis. Naked eye appearances can be misleading and because gastritis may be focal, biopsy may miss abnormal mucosa.

N.B. Beware of ascribing symptoms to gastritis — look for other causes of dyspepsia, etc.

Other tests may be indicated in many cases — Serum B_{12}, plasma gastrin, parietal cell and intrinsic factor antibodies, acid secretory studies and a B_{12} absorption test (e.g. Schilling test).

Treatment

Symptomatic patients with intestinal metaplasia or gastric atrophy may need to be screened long term because of the risk of developing gastric carcinoma.

DUODENITIS

Most but not all would agree that it is a variant of DU. Diagnosis is made by upper GI endoscopy with biopsy. Symptoms and treatment are the same as DU.

NON–ULCER DYSPEPSIA

Also called functional or nervous dyspepsia. The cause is unknown but it may be an abnormality of gastro-duodenal motility. It is considered by some to be part of the irritable bowel syndrome.

Symptoms and signs

Similar to DU although night pain is not a feature. Patients may have associated IBS or psychogenic vomiting and may describe exacerbation of symptoms at times of stress.

Investigation

Upper GI endoscopy, to exclude other causes of dyspepsia.

Diagnosis

By exclusion

Treatment

1. Explanation and reassurance
2. Regular meals
3. Avoid alcohol and smoking
4. Antacids with or without sedatives

In difficult cases, metoclopramide to improve gastroduodenal motility and an antidepressant may be indicated.

PROBLEMS AFTER GASTRIC SURGERY

Most may follow either vagotomy and a drainage operation or the various forms of partial gastrectomy.

Recurrent ulcer

Most common after operation for DU. Recurrences after partial gastrectomy and gastroenterostomy are most likely at the stoma.

Symptoms
Epigastric pain (may or may not be dyspeptic), nausea, vomiting, weight loss and GI haemorrhage.

Diagnosis and investigation
1. Upper GI endoscopy with biopsy.
2. Hollander test (to test completeness of vagotomy) — if patient has had previous vagotomy.
3. Serum calcium; plasma gastrin.

Treatment
1. Surgery — for most cases.
2. H_2 receptor antagonist — may be indicated in incompletely vagotomised patients.

Afferent loop syndrome

This is seen after Polya (Billroth II) gastric resections. Two types:
1. *Bloating and abdominal pain* 0.5–1 hour after eating is often followed by nausea and vomiting which may ease the pain. Vomit contains copious bile. The cause is incomplete emptying from the afferent loop of secretions provoked by eating. Barium studies may or may not show abnormalities. Plain abdominal X-ray at the time of symptoms may show obstructed loop. Diagnosis is usually made after careful history. Treatment is surgery.
2. *Bacterial overgrowth* in the afferent loop leading to a stagnant loop syndrome (see Ch. 10, p. 70). Treatment can be medical in the short term but surgical revision is the treatment of choice.

Dumping syndrome

Two types:
1. *Early* — occurs within 30 minutes of eating and is probably caused by rapid emptying of hyperosmolar gastric contents into the proximal small intestine leading to fluid shift into the gut lumen.

Symptoms — weakness, palpitations, tachycardia, dizziness, lightheadedness, drowsiness, abdominal distension and later abdominal cramps and diarrhoea.

2. *Late* — occurs 1.5–3 hours after eating and is caused by hypoglycaemia which results from insulin secretion in response to rapid increase in blood sugar secondary to rapid emptying of sugar containing foods into the small intestine. *Symptoms* — are those of hypoglycaemia, with weakness, faintness, anxiety, nausea, palpitations, hunger and are relieved by sugar.

Diagnosis

Both types are diagnosed by a careful history. Hypoglycaemia may be demonstrated by a 3 hour oral glucose tolerance test.

Treatment

Both forms are helped by frequent small dry meals with carbohydrate intake limited to 50 g/day. Surgical revision may be necessary for patients incapacitated by symptoms.

Bile reflux

Bile reflux gastritis, alkaline oesophageal reflux and bilious vomiting are probably part of the same syndrome of bile reflux into the stomach. However most patients with a partial gastrectomy have gastritis, usually around the stoma, with no symptoms.

Symptoms

Symptoms of gastritis with early satiety, epigastric pain, etc.; of oesophageal reflux with heartburn, regurgitation; of bilious vomiting.

Investigations

1. Upper GI endoscopy and biopsy — shows gastritis and bile in stomach.
2. BIDA scan — demonstrates bile reflux into the stomach and oesophagus.

Diagnosis

Upper GI endoscopy and history.

Treatment

1. Symptomatic measures for gastritis, vomiting or gastro–oesophageal reflux. Metoclopramide (lO mg tds) may be useful as it promotes gastric emptying and increases lower oesophageal sphincter pressure.
2. Bile salt binding agents — usually disappointing.
3. Bile diversion operation (e.g. Roux–en–Y anastomosis) — reserved for serious cases after adequate trial of medical therapy.

Nutritional and absorption disorders

Weight loss

This is common, especially after partial gastrectomy. Causes are poor dietary intake with or without steatorrhoea. Other causes of weight loss (see p. 8) must be excluded. Treatment — supervision and dietary advice.

Steatorrhoea

This is common after vagotomy and drainage and after Polya gastrectomy; and less common after Billroth I gastrectomy or highly selective vagotomy. It is usually mild and is rarely symptomatic. If symptoms occur, exclude other causes, especially bacterial overgrowth (see Ch. 10, p. 70). Mild steatorrhoea may be ignored. If symptomatic and no other cause is found — low fat diet and regular small meals. Pancreatic supplements may help difficult cases.

Metabolic bone disease

1. *Osteomalacia* — may follow partial gastrectomy; it is rare after vagotomy. It results from vitamin D and calcium malabsorption. Symptoms are bone pain and weakness. Diagnosis is suggested by low serum calcium, raised serum alkaline phosphatase, and low serum phosphate and is confirmed by bone biopsy or by bone X-ray (only abnormal in severe cases). Serum 25–OH–vitamin D is useful screening test for vitamin D deficiency. Treatment is calcium and vitamin D supplements for life.

2. *Osteoporosis* — common after partial gastrectomy, is diagnosed on bone X-ray (especially the spine) and is difficult to treat.

Anaemia

This is quite common after gastric resection but is rare after vagotomy.

1. *Iron deficiency* — most common type; is secondary to blood loss, iron malabsorption and/or poor intake.

2. B_{12} deficiency — usually results from decreased intrinsic factor production after gastric resection, or from bacterial overgrowth.

3. *Folate deficiency* — rarest; results from folate malabsorption and/or poor intake.

4. *Dimorphic* — mixture of iron and B_{12} deficiency anaemia; iron deficiency masks megaloblastosis.

Investigations

1. Full blood count, blood film and, sometimes, bone marrow

2. Serum iron, B_{12}; red cell folate

3. B_{12} absorption test (e.g. Schilling test) if B_{12} deficiency is present.

4. Exclude other causes of deficiency anaemia.

Treatment
Appropriate supplements for life; probably all patients with partial gastrectomies should have prophylactic iron supplements for life.

Pulmonary tuberculosis

Gastric surgery is a risk factor for pulmonary TB; it should be considered in patients who are losing weight.

Carcinoma

There is an increased risk of gastric carcinoma 10 years or more after partial gastrectomy.

Post–vagotomy diarrhoea

This is common after truncal vagotomy and is often associated with dumping. Diarrhoea may be related to steatorrhoea but in most cases, no cause is found. The mechanism is uncertain but may be related to motility disturbances and/or bile salt malabsorption. It is necessary to exclude steatorrhoea and other causes of diarrhoea (see later). Treatment is with anti-diarrhoeal agents (e.g. codeine phosphate) but a high fibre diet may help some patients. Dietary treatment for associated dumping (see earlier) may help. Some patients respond to cholestyramine.

GASTRIC CARCINOMA

Deaths about 12 000/year (England and Wales) but prevalence is declining. Rare before 30 years of age and commonest in 60 to 70 year olds. Male : Female ratio is 2 : 1.

Risk factors
These may include diet (rice, smoked foods, nitrosamines), pernicious anaemia and gastric atrophy, gastritis, gastric surgery, gastric polyps. Benign GU is probably not a risk factor. There may be a family history of gastric carcinoma and the disorder is commoner in people with blood Group A.

Sites
Pylorus and antrum (50–60%), body (20–30%), cardia (5–20%). Carcinoma after partial gastrectomy tends to occur at the stoma.

Pathology
Macroscopic — fungating, ulcerating, diffusely infiltrative, superficial spreading, linitis plastica.

Microscopic
Virtually all are adenocarcinomas of the following types: papillomatous

carcinoma, adenocarcinoma, carcinoma simplex, colloid carcinoma, scirrhous carcinoma, anaplastic carcinoma.

Symptoms
Weight loss, epigastric pain, nausea and vomiting, haematemesis, anorexia, dysphagia, eructation, regurgitation, early satiety, malaise, weakness, fever.

Signs
Epigastric mass (30–50%), palpable left supraclavicular lymph node (Virchow's node) (5%), weight loss, hepatomegaly, anaemia, secondary tumour in pouch of Douglas on rectal examination.

Metastases
Adjacent organs, peritoneum, lymph nodes, liver, lungs, bone.

Complications
The most important is obstruction.

Diagnosis

1. Barium meal — double contrast — frequently suggests the diagnosis; may be the only way to diagnose linitis plastica.
2. Upper GI endoscopy with brush cytology and biopsy — necessary in all cases to provide histological proof of carcinoma and its type, to check suspicious lesions and healed ulcers (ulcerating gastric carcinomas can temporarily heal with cimetidine) and to assess the extent of the tumour. It is easy to miss early lesions and linitis plastica.

Treatment

1. *Surgery* — resection provides only hope of cure; subtotal resection rather than total gastrectomy is usually possible and has a lower mortality; palliative resection is indicated to prevent obstruction in cases with metastases.
2. *Chemotherapy* — various regimes have been tried with some short term improvement in survival; 5-fluorouracil is the most widely used chemotherapeutic agent.
3. *Radiotherapy* — most gastric carcinomas are *not* radio sensitive.
4. *Medical palliation* — endoscopic intubation of obstructing carcinoma (especially at the fundus) in patients with metastases may prevent complete obstruction.

Prognosis

Overall 5–10% 5 year survival; curative resection has about 25% 5 year survival; virtually no patients treated with palliation alone will survive 5 years.

EARLY GASTRIC CARCINOMA

This is carcinoma confined to the mucosa and submucosa. It is increasingly recognized, particularly in Japan, and in Europe it makes up 5% of all gastric carcinomas. There may be no symptoms until the mucosa ulcerates causing dyspeptic symptoms. It is easy to miss an early carcinoma endoscopically — therefore all unusual, suspicious or localised mucosal lesions should be biopsied. Diagnosis is made by brush cytology and biopsy via the endoscope although double contrast barium meal can demonstrate the lesions. Survival rates of >90% at 5 years after curative resection have been achieved in Japan.

9. GASTROINTESTINAL HAEMORRHAGE

UPPER GASTROINTESTINAL HAEMORRHAGE

Causes of overt GI haemorrhage and important aspects of the history have been discussed earlier (Ch. 3).

Examination

This is rarely helpful in pinpointing the source of the bleed. However, the following should not be missed:
1. Rectal examination.
2. Cutaneous signs, e.g. jaundice, stigmata of chronic liver disease, telangiectasia, oral pigmentation of Peutz–Jegher's syndrome, manifestations of a bleeding diathesis.
3. Signs of severe haemorrhage — pallor, thirst, sweating, cold peripheries, agitation, faintness, confusion, hypotension, postural hypotension, tachycardia.
4. Signs of any other disease which may increase the risk to the patient, especially chronic cardiac and respiratory disorders.

Initial Management

Admission to hospital is mandatory, however trivial the bleed appears to be. Except perhaps for patients with minor bleeds (especially if young), all patients should be nursed in an intensive nursing area or an ITU.
1. Ensure adequate airway; give oxygen if the patient is restless or shocked.
2. I.v. infusion (see later); CVP line if the patient is shocked.
3. Blood for cross–match (at least two units, even if the bleed seems trivial), full blood count, prothrombin time, urea, electrolytes, liver function tests; measure blood gases in shocked patients.
4. Give sedation, if patient is anxious (e.g. diazepam 5–10 mg i.v.) but remember agitation may be a sign of shock or continued bleeding; beware of opiates because of their emetic effect and avoid all sedatives especially opiates or

barbiturates, in patients with chronic liver disease and/or jaundice.

5. Cimetidine is *not* indicated until a definite diagnosis has been made.

6. Wide bore nasogastric tube — while mandatory in USA, in UK it is probably only indicated in severe haemorrhage as it can cause erosions or disturb clot and is unpleasant for the patient. It should only be passed after the diagnosis has been made. The patient feels more comfortable without blood in the stomach and regular aspiration is indicated if bleeding is continuing, has stopped or has restarted.

7. Pass urinary catheter, if the patient is shocked.

8. Other measures:
   a. Vitamin K (10 mg i.v.), if the patient is jaundiced or if chronic liver disease is suspected
   b. Treat any other disease which may be present, e.g. heart failure.

Intravenous infusion

Initially give normal saline; but if the patient is shocked, give a plasma expander, e.g. plasma protein solution, albumin, or dextran 70 (can interfere with cross–matching) until blood arrives. Rarely uncross–matched O negative blood may be necessary. For all large transfusions: use whole blood, warm blood to 37°C, use blood filters, change the giving set every 5–6 units and give calcium gluconate 10% 10 ml i.v., fresh frozen plasma one unit and platelet concentrate one unit for every 10 units of blood transfused.

Monitoring of progress

Blood pressure, pulse and in severe cases, urine output and CVP as well as haemoglobin and haematocrit. Blood loss is often more than is apparent from the clinical state of the patient (especially in young patients). Continued bleeding is indicated by sweating, agitation, hyperactive bowel sounds, tachycardia, hypotension. Remember melaena may be present up to five days after a single upper GI tract bleed and faecal occult blood may remain positive for up to two weeks after a bleed.

Severe haemorrhagic shock

The patient requires oxygen, CVP line, urinary catheterization and urgent blood volume replacement monitored by CVP and urine output. Blood gases should be measured as hypoxia will impair recovery and requires appropriate treatment; metabolic acidosis indicates severe shock.

1. If CVP and urinary output are high, the patient is being over transfused and therefore, the transfusion rate should be reduced.

2. If CVP and urinary output is low either (a) or (b):
   a. Cardiac output is normal and renal function is impaired; therefore give osmotic diuretic (e.g. mannitol 25 g i.v.) or,

if no response, give loop diuretic (e.g. frusemide 250 mg i.v.).

b. Cardiac output is impaired — exclude myocardial infarction by ECG then give dopamine infusion (2.5 μg/kg/min titrated to response). Remember in large transfusions, citrate toxicity may cause myocardial depression therefore consider giving calcium gluconate 10% 10 ml i.v.

Diagnosis (see Part 1)

The most important investigation is upper GI endoscopy, which should be performed within 12–18 hours of admission. If endoscopy is delayed longer, the diagnostic yield rapidly falls off. Endoscopy very early after admission is rarely practical in every case but it should be performed in patients with severe haemorrhage in whom early surgery is contemplated.

Further management

Variceal haemorrhage
See Ch 12, Section on 'PORTAL HYPERTENSION'

Non-variceal haemorrhage
General measures after diagnosis:

1. Notify surgical colleagues and take decisions jointly.
2. Monitor for signs of rebleeding or continued bleeding.
3. Bed rest until the bleeding has stopped.
4. Free fluids are safe after bleed provided investigations or surgery are not contemplated; a light diet can be started when the bleeding has stopped and patient does not feel nauseated.
5. Prevention of rebleed — a number of therapies has been suggested, e.g. vasopressin infusion, gastric hypothermia, tranexamic acid, somatostatin, H_2 blockers but there is no general agreement as to their value and they are not indicated routinely.

Examples of non-variceal haemorrhage

Chronic peptic ulcer
GI haemorrhage occurs at sometime in 20–30% of patients referred to hospital with peptic ulcer and 80–90% of patients have a previous dyspeptic history. The risk of rebleeding is greater in the first 48 hours and in patients who present with haematemesis, who have a large initial bleed (with shock), who have a GU rather than a DU and whose ulcer at endoscopy shows active bleeding, adherent clot or visible vessel in ulcer. Mortality is related particularly to rebleeding and to age and is much higher in GU than DU (16% v 9%).

Treatment

1. Initial measures
2. Investigations.
3. General measures.
4. H_2 receptor blockers — should be started as soon as the diagnosis is made and given by mouth as soon as the bleeding stops.
5. Indications for surgery — every patient with peptic ulcer should have surgery before they need 10 or more units of blood over 72 hours.
    a. *Duodenal ulcer* — under 60 years of age, surgery is indicated for active bleeding (at endoscopy), rebleed or history of previous bleed. Over 60 years of age, especially if some coexistent disease is present, early surgery is indicated for continued bleeding.
    b. *Gastric ulcer* — surgery is indicated if the ulcer is large and/or deep, if stigmata of bleeding are present, if there is a rebleed and if there is a history of previous bleed.
    c. *Post surgical peptic ulcer* — treat as GU.
6. Other interventional therapy — various endoscopic coagulation techniques with lasers, bipolar electrodes, thermal probes etc. are being evaluated but as yet none are available outside a few specialist centres. Interventional radiology, where bleeding vessels are embolised at angiography, has a role in severe bleeding in the elderly or infirm who are too ill for surgery.

Acute peptic ulcer and erosions

Most cases stop with simple supportive therapy. H_2 receptor blockers with or without regular antacids are usually given. In the few cases that continue to bleed, vasopression infusion or oral tranexamic acid may stop the bleeding. Rarely, surgery may be necessary because of continued bleeding despite active medical treatment. Full coagulation screen must be checked in patients with severe or continued bleeding.

Stress ulcer

These are more common in patients with severe disorders of other systems and they often bleed. Full coagulation screen must be checked and any abnormalities corrected if possible. Treatment initially is supportive with H_2 receptor blockers and antacids. Unfortunately surgery may be necessary if bleeding continues but has a high mortality because of associated disease.

Mallory–Weiss syndrome

Although the history may be typical, diagnosis must be confirmed at endoscopy. Most cases settle with supportive therapy only. If bleeding continues vasopressin infusion may be tried but if all else fails, surgery may be necessary.

Reflux oesophagitis

Rarely causes more than a minor haemorrhage which settles with supportive therapy, H_2 receptor blockers and regular antacids. Patient should be nursed at 45° to minimize reflux. Surgery is very rarely necessary acutely.

Oesophageal (or Barrett's) ulcer

This ulcer in the distal oesophagus is usually seen in the elderly and can cause severe haemorrhage. Medical therapy with H_2 receptor blockers etc may be successful, but surgery may be indicated although can be difficult and has a high mortality.

Gastric ulcer in a hiatal hernia

Treat as any other GU. Early surgery is often neccesary but any procedure must include a hiatal hernia repair.

LOWER GASTROINTESTINAL HAEMORRHAGE

Clinical aspects, causes and diagnosis have been discussed (Ch. 3). Initial management is the same as for upper GI haemorrhage. Bleeding nearly always stops spontaneously and specific treatment depends on the cause. However, in continued bleeding, vasopressin infusion may stop bleeding.

10. SMALL AND LARGE BOWEL DISEASE

MALABSORPTION

Causes

See Chapter 5

Symptoms and signs

Malabsorption is not a disease but a symptom of disease. It is a syndrome, of extremely variable severity, which may be caused by any one of a large number of diseases each of which may have its own characteristic symptom pattern. However, symptoms of any form of malabsorption may include diarrhoea, weakness, fatigue, malaise, abdominal distension, pain and rumbling as well as specific symptoms related to a particular deficiency (see below). Non specific signs include pigmentation, wasting, abdominal distension, loud borborygmi, finger clubbing. The syndrome of malabsorption per se presents in one of three ways:

1. *Asymptomatically*
   Accidental finding of features suggesting malabsorption in a patient undergoing investigation of unrelated problems, e.g. finding of a mixed deficiency anaemia on a routine blood film.

2. *Acute malabsorption syndrome*
   Characteristically presents with weight loss and diarrhoea. Steatorrhoea is invariably present but when severe the features of steatorrhoea are often masked by the high water content of the stool (i.e. diarrhoea). Symptoms are of relatively sudden onset, often with a recognisable 'trigger' event, e.g. recent surgery (such as vagotomy, cholecystectomy), antibiotic induced diarrhoea, episode of pancreatitis or infection.

3. *Insidious malabsorption*
   Now by far the commonest presentation. Weight loss can be absent, small and not noticed. Small and constipated stools

can contain gross fat. Patient can present to any hospital department with deficiency symptoms caused by malabsorption.

Examples include:

Anaemia — iron, folate, B_{12} or mixed deficiencies

Skin rashes — dermatitis herpetiformis

Aphthous ulceration and glossitis

Oedema — hypoproteinaemia

Metabolic bone disease — Vitamin D deficiency and osteoporosis

Bleeding tendency — hypoprothrombinaemia

Renal tract calculi — hyperoxaluria

Neuropathies and myopathies

Diabetes mellitus — pancreatic disease

Growth impairment

Amenorrhoea, infertility

Diagnosis

Two stages are required:

1. *Is malabsorption present?*
   Because most diseases which cause malabsorption will interfere with the absorption of fat, the detection of steatorrhoea is the crucial first stage in answering this question. When there is a clinical suspicion of malabsorption, perform a three day faecal fat balance. Other tests for steatorrhoea, e.g. ^{14}C–triolein test, do not indicate the severity of the steatorrhoea but are useful in screening. Other screening tests for malabsorption are unreliable, but probably the best is measurement of red cell folate levels.
2. *What is the disease causing the malabsorption?*
   Because the number of diseases which may produce malabsorption is so large, a logical sequence of investigation is recommended as below.

Investigations

Investigations in a patient with proven malabsorption are designed:

1. To indicate the consequences the malabsorptive state so that treatment can commence — e.g. measurement of iron, folate and B_{12} levels so that anaemias may be appropriately treated, measurement of prothrombin time to assess parenteral Vitamin K requirement, calcium and alkaline phosphatase estimation as assessment of Vitamin D deficiency.
2. To diagnose the disease causing the malabsorption. The likely cause or site of disease causing the malabsorption is often

indicated by the history and physical examination — e.g. pancreatic disease is the commonest cause of malabsorption in patients known to abuse alcohol. But if there are no real pointers to the cause in a patient then two investigations will reveal the cause of malabsorption in most cases — barium follow-through and jejunal biopsy.

Barium follow-through (Small bowel meal)

This examines the gross anatomy of the small intestine. Diseases amenable to diagnosis on barium follow-through include:

       Intestinal fistulae and resections
       Intestinal strictures
       Jejunal diverticulosis
       Systemic sclerosis
       Crohn's disease
       Lymphoma

N.B. In many diffuse, small intestinal disorders causing malabsorption — e.g. coeliac disease, tropical sprue, Whipple's disease, the barium follow-through may show only the non-specific 'malabsorption' pattern.

Jejunal biopsy

This examines the microscopic anatomy of the small intestine.

   Diseases amenable to diagnosis on jejunal biopsy are those causing diffuse mucosal damage and include

       Coeliac disease (and dermatitis herpetiformis)
       Crohn's disease
       Intestinal lymphangiectasia
       Immunodeficiency states
       Giardiasis
       Abetalipoproteinaemia
       Tropical sprue
       Radiation enteritis
       Amyloid
       Systemic sclerosis
       Whipple's disease.

If the gross anatomy and the microscopic anatomy of the small intestine are normal, then the likely site of disease causing malabsorption is the pancreas. Remember that 80% or more of the gland must be damaged before malabsorption and steatorrhoea occur. Early or mild pancreatic disease can be difficult to detect, but little significant pancreatic disease would be missed after:

     1. Anatomical assessment of the pancreas by:
       — plain abdominal film for calcification
       — ultrasonic scan
       — endoscopic retrograde pancreatography

2. Functional assessment of the pancreas:
   — endocrine function by glucose tolerance test
   — exocrine function by secretin/pancreozymin stimulation
       test, Lundh test, or one of the tubeless tests (such as
       NBT PABA or fluorescein dilaurate).

Syndromes of isolated or specific malabsorption, if suspected, need
appropriate specific investigations e.g. pernicious anaemia (Schilling test),
alactasia (see below), SI bacterial overgrowth (see below), bile salt
malabsorption ^{14}C-glycocholate breath test; ^{75}SeHCAT test), ileal
dysfunction (Schilling test; ^{75}SeHCAT test). Some forms of malabsorption,
e.g. in thyrotoxicosis, defy classification but the diagnosis is often fairly
obvious.

Treatment

Treatment should be directed at:
1. The consequences of malabsorption — This is particularly
   important in those cases of malabsorption in which there is
   no specific treatment of the cause and in which the
   accompanying protein losing enteropathy can be severe, e.g.
   intestinal lymphangiectasia, amyloid, etc.
2. The specific disease which is causing the malabsorption, e.g.
   Crohn's disease, coeliac disease, etc.

General management of the effects of malabsorption

Diet
High protein, high calorie but low fat diet — symptoms of steatorrhoea
are exacerbated by dietary fat. Medium chain triglycerides which are
better absorbed than normal dietary fats are a very useful source of
calories and usually well tolerated in patients with steatorrhoea.

Clotting defects
Usually due to Vitamin K malabsorption. Correct with intramuscular
phytomenadione.

Metabolic bone disease
Usually osteomalacia. Correct established osteomalacia with 1 μg daily of
l-alphahydroxycholecalciferol or 50 000u calciferol weekly.

Anaemia
Commonly due to folate deficiency with or without iron deficiency. Oral
folic acid 10 mg tds and ferrous gluconate 300 mg tds usually suffice.
Beware of Vitamin B_{12} deficiency in ileal disease (e.g. Crohn's disease,
extensive coeliac disease) and correct with intramuscular
hydroxocobalamin 1000 μg monthly.

Management of specific diseases: See relevant section

COELIAC DISEASE

Damage to the small intestine is caused by dietary gluten (from wheat, barley, rye and in some individuals, oats); the mechanism is uncertain (possibly immunological). It is often associated with tissue types HLA-B8 and HLA-DW3. The exact prevalence is unknown; estimates for UK are 1:1100, West of Ireland 1:300; first degree relatives of coeliac patients 1:10

Pathology: sub total villous atrophy of the small intestinal mucosa
Clinical features: it presents at any age but especially in infancy and early adult life. Asymptomatic cases are found and presentation may be precipitated by infection, surgery, pregnancy etc. Clinical features are those of malabsorption (see earlier) or of the complications of coeliac disease e.g. small bowel ulceration, neuropathy, vasculitis or non-Hodgkin's lymphoma.
Associated disorders: dermatitis herpetiformis, diabetes mellitus, autoimmune and atopic diseases, fibrosing alveolitis.
Investigations: see malabsorption; jejunal biopsy is mandatory.
Diagnosis: subtotal villous atrophy of the SI which recovers on a gluten free diet.
Treatment: A gluten free diet for life and nutritional supplements are given as indicated. Constipation is sometimes a problem and may benefit from rice bran. Secondary lactase deficiency may require lactose restriction. Corticosteroids may be indicated in symptomatic non-responders. Repeat jejunal biopsy after 3–6 months on the diet is vital.
Prognosis: all children and 90% (or more) of adults respond clinically and morphologically to the diet; occasional non-responders are seen. Malignancy should be considered in non-responders or in patients with unexplained deterioration. Other reasons for apparent non response are non-compliance, intestinal ulceration, lactase deficiency.

LACTASE DEFICIENCY (ALACTASIA)

There are 3 types of SI brush border lactase deficiency: primary (progressive loss of enzyme activity after early childhood; normal outside northern Europe; seen in 5–10% of Britons); secondary (caused by SI mucosal damage e.g. coeliac disease), congenital (very rare). The result is lactose malabsorption which may cause diarrhoea, flatulence and abdominal swelling, rumbling and discomfort. It is diagnosed by measuring lactase activity in a jejunal biopsy. Useful indirect tests (assess lactose absorption) are the lactose breath hydrogen test (correlates well with lactase activity except in some patients with SI mucosal damage or with gastric or intestinal surgery) and the lactose tolerance test (relatively inaccurate). Alactasia is treated by reducing lactose intake until symptoms are relieved.

SMALL INTESTINAL BACTERIAL OVERGROWTH

This is seen in the elderly or in patients with structural SI abnormalities e.g. strictures, fistulae, bypassed loops, diverticula. The result is the stagnant (blind) loop syndrome with malabsorption (see earlier). Jejunal juice aspiration (with aerobic *and* anaerobic culture) makes the diagnosis (abnormal colony count >10^6/ml). The best indirect test is the glucose breath hydrogen test. Other such tests are the ^{14}C-glycocholate breath test or the Schilling test (before and after antibiotics) but these are also abnormal with ileal dysfunction. Treatment is with antibiotics (e.g. tetracycline, metronidazole), which may have to be repeated regularly, and surgical revision of any structural disorder if possible.

INFLAMMATORY BOWEL DISEASE

An all-embracing term for the idiopathic chronic inflammatory disorders of the intestine, ulcerative colitis and Crohn's disease (regional enteritis).

Ulcerative colitis and Crohn's colitis

Ulcerative colitis is a chronic relapsing mucosal inflammatory disorder of unknown aetiology; Crohn's colitis may be differentiated from ulcerative colitis by mucosal appearance, histology, radiological appearances, patchiness of the lesion, rectal sparing and perianal disease (tags, fissures, fistulae) but in practice it is often difficult. Management is similar for both disorders and perhaps only in terms of prognosis is a definite diagnosis necessary.

Symptoms — bloody diarrhoea and abdominal pain which is often eased by defaecation; in severe cases, nausea, vomiting, abdominal distension and fever; symptoms of complications (see later).

Signs — often none; colonic tenderness; in severe cases, fever, anaemia, tachycardia, abdominal distension, tenderness and even peritonism; signs of complications.

Investigations
1. Stool observation, microscopy and culture.
2. Perianal inspection.
3. Sigmoidoscopy — gently especially in severely ill patients.
4. Rectal biopsy — unless patient is severely ill.
5. Blood tests: full blood count; differential WCC, ESR or viscosity, acute phase proteins, e.g. orosomucoids, C-reactive protein, blood urea and electrolytes, serum proteins, liver function tests, serum iron and TIBC (or transferrin).

6. Radiology:
   a. Barium enema (double contrast) unless patient is very ill.
   b. Plain abdominal X-ray — if patient is very ill.
7. Colonoscopy — only indicated in cases of diagnostic difficulty and not if the patient is very ill.
8. Tests of SI function — may be indicated if associated small intestinal disease is suspected.

Diagnosis

Typical histological features of ulcerative or Crohn's colitis on large bowel biopsy. *N.B.* Rectal sparing occurs in Crohn's colitis; non–specific histology does not exclude Crohn's colitis; colonic infection *must* be excluded; colinic mucosa may look normal but be abnormal histologically in Crohn's colitis.

Management and treatment

Aims of treatment

As the only curative therapy in ulcerative colitis is panproctocolectomy, the aim is to keep the patient symptom free, to suppress inflammatory activity and if it is troublesome, to prevent relapses and to screen for and treat complications.

Follow up

Life long — even for ulcerative colitis patients with a panproctocolectomy who are at risk of mechanical, metabolic and psychological problems and of prestomal ileitis.

Assessment

1. Inflammatory activity: symptoms and signs, sigmoidoscopy and biopsy, haemoglobin, WCC, serum albumin, acute phase proteins.
2. Extent of disease: barium enema (double contrast), or colonoscopy and biopsy. Patients may have total colitis at the onset or may have subtotal, left sided or distal colitis, or proctitis. Patients without total colitis will need regular assessment to monitor progression.
   N.B. — Barium studies may underestimate the extent of colitis.

Treatment

Is the same, whether the patient presents with colitis *de novo* or with a flare up of known colitis. Treatment depends on severity rather than extent of disease.

Severe colitis

Severe bloody diarrhoea, nausea, vomiting, abdominal distension and tenderness (with or without rebound), fever, dehydration, anaemia, tachycardia; it is confirmed by anaemia, elevated acute phase proteins, neutrophilia and hypoalbuminaemia.

Initial management
1. Admit; complete bed rest, nil by mouth.
2. Gentle sigmoidoscopy with minimal air to confirm diagnosis, no rectal biopsy.
3. Plain abdominal X-ray — to assess degree of colonic dilatation and presence or absence of perforation; avoid barium enema.
4. Intravenous infusion — replace fluid and electrolytes (especially potassium); transfuse up to haemoglobin of 13–14 g%; parenteral nutrition is not indicated unless the patient is very malnourished.
5. Nasogastric tube — only if patient is vomiting.
6. Prednisolone 60-80 mg i.v. (or equivalent dose of hydrocortisone).
7. Parenteral antibiotics (including cover for faecal anaerobes) — for severe cases, or if there is colonic dilatation.
8. Notify GI surgical team — management decisions should be made jointly by physicians and surgeons.

   N.B. There is no place for therapy with sulphasalazine azathioprine, antidiarrhoeals, antispasmodics or for therapy per rectum. A major risk in severe colitis is the development of toxic megacolon, therefore:

   a. Avoid — Opiates (antidiarrhoeals, analgesics), rectal biopsy, barium enema, steroid enemas.
   b. Treat — Hypokalaemia
   c. Monitor — Abdominal girth
   Plain abdominal X–ray

Daily assessment
Full examination, check temperature and pulse chart, abdominal girth, abdominal X-ray, haemoglobin, urea, electrolytes, joint medical/surgical consultation, check for DVT (increased risk in colitis).

Indications for surgery
1. Progessive deterioration (acute fulminating colitis).
2. Toxic megacolon (it is controversial whether it is a relative or an absolute indication).
3. Perforation.
4. No change after 24–48 hours medical treatment. If in doubt, *operate* — delay leads to rapidly increasing mortality.
5. Relapse when feeding restarts after an apparent good response to 5–7 days of intensive medical therapy.

Continued medical management
Recovery indicated by symptomatic improvement, loss of fever, decreased pulse rate, loss of abdominal tenderness and distension; blood tests return to normal more slowly. After 5–7 days — stop antibiotics. Give steroids orally — progressively reduce dose of prednisolone 2.5–5 mg/day every 3–4 days to a dose of 20 mg/day at discharge.

Moderate colitis

Bloody diarrhoea, abdominal discomfort; possibly nausea, fever; haematological and biochemical signs of activity.

Treatment

Admit for for bed rest, however, some cases could be managed as outpatients provided they can be seen frequently.

1. Full clinical, haematological and biochemical assessment; plain abdominal X–ray.
2. Prednisolone 20–40 mg/day by mouth (i.v. if nauseated)
3. Sulphasalazine 3–4 g/day (in divided doses) — some patients may respond to this alone.
4. High calorie, high protein diet.
5. Transfuse if anaemic; give iron by mouth if indicated.
6. Give steroid enemas if there are severe rectal symptoms.

Mild colitis

Diarrhoea, often bloody, with little other upset, little or no haematological or biochemical evidence of activity.

Treatment

Most cases are treated as outpatients. Antidiarrhoeal agents may help. Give iron (if indicated), sulphasalazine 3–4 g/day and steroid retention enemas; oral steroids are usually not indicated.

Treatment between exacerbations

1. Regular reassurance, support and encouragement.
2. Prednisolone — no value in maintaining remissions, therefore try to reduce dose and stop; patients who relapse on dose reductions or after cessation of treatment may require very slow dosage reduction; some patients (especially with Crohn's colitis) may need continued therapy to suppress inflammatory activity — try to keep dose below 10 mg/day to minimize side effects.
3. Sulphasalazine — of proven value in reducing the number of relapses in ulcerative colitis; no evidence that it does the same in Crohn's colitis but is usually given as maintenance nevertheless (dose 2–3 g/day); high incidence of side effects (1–5%); new preparations without the sulphapyridine component are becoming available e.g. mesalazine
4. Azathioprine — no value in maintenance but can be used as a 'steroid sparing' agent and in the treatment of patients failing to settle on steroids alone; be wary of its use because of its potentially serious side effects.
5. Haematinics — watch for iron deficiency in all cases and folate deficiency in those on sulphasalazine; Crohn's colitis patients with associated small bowel disease may have folate

and/or B_{12} deficiency, therefore treat with appropriate
supplements.
6. Diet — no definite rules but many patients find a high fibre
   diet makes them more comfortable.

If patients with inactive colonic disease have continued diarrhoea,
consider lactose intolerance, small intestinal disease (in Crohn's colitis) or
associated irritable bowel syndrome.

Surgery in colitis

If possible, surgery should be performed electively but in certain
situations emergency colectomy is necessary.
1. Absolutely indicated — Acute fulminating colitis
                          Perforation
                          Carcinoma
2. Usually indicated — Toxic megacolon
                       Massive haemorrhage
3. Sometimes indicated — Persistently active disease
                         Perianal disease
                         Stricture
                         Arthritis
                         Pyoderma gangrenosum
                         Growth failure (children)

N.B. Patients with Crohn's colitis are more likely to have a
colectomy for persistent disease activity than patients with
ulcerative colitis.

The operation of choice is panproctocolectomy with ileostomy; ileorectal
anastomosis and colectomy is an alternative for patients with good rectal
capacity and no perianal disease. For some patients with ulcerative
colitis, the construction of an ileoanal pouch is an important development
in surgical management

Complication of colitis

See later

IDIOPATHIC PROCTITIS

1. Bloody diarrhoea with no systemic symptoms
2. Disease is limited to the rectum and distal sigmoid colon
3. In only 30% of patients does disease spread proximally
4. Histology usually shows non specific inflammatory changes,
   but Crohn's disease may be seen.

Treatment
Sulphasalazine acutely and as maintenance therapy and steroid retention
enemas acutely; some patients have a tendency to constipation and the

passage of hard stools can precipitate bleeding therefore in these cases treat constipation (see earlier) as well as rectal inflammation.

CROHN'S DISEASE OF THE SMALL INTESTINE

This is a chronic relapsing mucosal and submucosal granulomatous inflammatory disorder of unknown aetiology. It can occur anywhere in the small intestine but is commonest in the terminal ileum. It often occurs with Crohn's colitis. It heals by fibrosis, can recur proximally or distally from the site of first involvement and has a tendency to form fistulae.

Symptoms
Diarrhoea (with or without features of steatorrhoea), central abdominal colic and/or right iliac fossa pain, fever, anorexia, weight loss, malaise; associated malabsorption or complications may lead to other symptoms; onset may be acute or insidious.

Signs
Right iliac fossa tenderness, rebound tenderness or palpable mass can be found. Often there are none.

Investigations
1. Stool inspection, microscopy and culture.
2. Perianal inspection, sigmoidoscopy and biopsy.
3. Blood tests — FBC, acute phase proteins, blood urea and electrolytes, serum calcium, magnesium, and 25-hydroxyvitamin D, serum proteins, liver function tests, serum iron, TIBC (or transferrin), serum B_{12}, red cell (or serum) folate
4. Radiology — barium follow through or small bowel enema
5. Other tests (as indicated):
   For malabsorption — three day faecal fat
   For ileal dysfunction — Schilling test, bile acid absorption tests, e.g. ^{14}C glycocholate breath test
   For bacterial overgrowth — glucose breath hydrogen test or jejunal/ileal juice aspiration
   To exclude Yersiniosis — Yersinia antibodies
   In diffuse SI Crohn's disease — Jejunal biopsy (to exclude coeliac disease, etc.)

Diagnosis
Most cases are initially diagnosed on characteristic radiological features; firm histological diagnosis can only be made when affected gut is resected or if there is associated histologically proven colonic Crohn's disease. Acute ileitis may be caused by infections, e.g. Yersiniosis, and diffuse Crohn's jejuno–ileitis may be difficult to separate from other diffuse

small intestinal disease causing malabsorption (e.g. coeliac disease) without jejunal biopsy.

Management

Aims of treatment, follow-up and assessment of inflammatory activity are the same as for colitis (see earlier).

Treatment

This can usually be done in the outpatients clinic. Indications for admission are severe diarrhoea, weight loss and malnutrition, obstruction or systemic ill health.

1. Regular reassurance, support and encouragement.
2. Diet — high protein, high calorie; some patients feel more comfortable on a high fibre diet but avoid roughage if patient has obstructive symptoms. There is no convincing evidence yet of a therapeutic benefit from high fibre, low refined carbohydrate diets or exclusion diets in Crohn's disease.
3. Haematinics — treat iron, B_{12} and folate deficiencies as they occur; and ill patients with a haemoglobin <10 g% need transfusion.
4. Antidiarrhoeal agents — e.g. codeine phosphate 30–60 mg tds or loperamide 2–4 mg tds.
5. Suppression of inflammatory activity — *N.B.* not all cases of Crohn's disease need steroids.
   a. mild cases — general and symptomatic treatment only.
   b. moderate cases — try sulphasalazine 3–4 g/day but if no response treat as a severe case.
   c. Severe cases — steroids, e.g. prednisolone 20–40 mg/day. They do not alter outcome or reduce risk of relapse therefore dose should be reduced or stopped when possible; however, this can be difficult as reduction in dose often causes relapse.
6. Azathioprine (controversial) — has some use as steroid sparing agent and it does benefit the occasional non-responder to steroids and heal the occasional long standing fistula; but beware of side effects, especially in young adults.
7. Antibiotics — are only indicated if abscess is present.
8. **Treatment of specific problems**
   a. Obstruction — if severe, admit for 'drip and suck'; patients rarely need emergency surgery. If sub-acute or less severe, give low residue diet. Obstruction may be due to either an inflammatory or a fibrotic stricture; if the former, treat with corticosteroids; if the latter, surgery will probably be needed when the acute episode has settled.
   b. Malnutrition — if severe, enteral nutrition (parenteral nutrition is rarely indicated).
   c. Malabsorption — replace malabsorbed nutrients, e.g.

folate, vitamins B_{12}, D, K. If the patient has steatorrhoea, start a low fat diet.

d. Blind loop syndrome — may be treated medically (with antibiotics, e.g. oxytetracycline, metronidazole) but surgery is usually indicated.

e. Bile salt malabsorption — seen in patients with ileal disease or resection; treat with cholestyramine or aluminium hydroxide gel.

f. Fistula — early postoperative fistulae may heal, but long standing postoperative or spontaneous fistulae usually require surgical excision of tract and of diseased bowel from which they arise; azathioprine or bowel rest with total parenteral nutrition can sometimes heal a long standing fistula.

9. **Surgery**
   a. Absolutely indicated — carcinoma, perforation
   b. Frequently indicated — fibrotic stricture, abscess, fistula, stagnant loop
   c. Sometimes indicated — localised active disease

The role of surgery is controversial particularly in the treatment of localised active disease because of the risk of recurrence and the danger of succeeding operations leading to the short bowel syndrome; both these worries are probably overemphasised.

COMPLICATIONS OF INFLAMMATORY BOWEL DISEASE

Local complications of colitis

1. *Perianal disease*
   Haemorrhoids — if troublesome, dilatation under general anaesthetic and avoid surgery
   Skin tags — ignore
   Perianal
       Abscess — early, use antibiotics
                 — late, use surgical drainage
       Fistula — ignore, lay open fistulous track or proctectomy
2. *Pseudopolyps* — no treatment necessary
3. *Toxic megacolon* — treat as for acute severe colitis; early surgery advisable.
4. *Carcinoma* — panproctocolectomy; screening for carcinoma is discussed later (p. 96).
5. *Massive haemorrhage* — supportive therapy but often requires surgery
6. *Strictures* — rarely require treatment in ulcerative colitis; may need excision in Crohn's colitis

Local complications of small intestinal Crohn's disease
Perforation, carcinoma and fistulae are discussed earlier

Systemic complications of inflammatory bowel disease

1. *Arthritis* — In Crohn's disease, it is relatively benign; treat with non steroidal anti-inflammatory drugs. In ulcerative colitis, arthritis can be severe and destructive requiring steroids and even panproctocolectomy.
2. *Skin disease*
   a. Erythema nodosum — none or non-steroidal anti-inflammatory drugs.
   b. Pyoderma gangrenosum — steroids or, in severe cases with colitis, panproctocolectomy
   c. Vasculitis of ulcerative colitis — steroids
3. *Other complications* — the following are treated in the same way as in non-IBD patients:
   a. Hepatobiliary disorders — fatty infiltration, sclerosing cholangitis, chronic active hepatitis, cirrhosis, bile duct carcinoma
   b. Cholelithiasis
   c. Renal diseases — pyelonephritis, ureteric obstruction, urinary calculi
   d. Amyloidosis
   e. Ocular disorders — iritis, episcleritis
   f. Thromboembolism

INTESTINAL ISCHAEMIA

Three important syndromes:

1. Acute intestinal failure (Acute intestinal ischaemia)

Commonly the result of ischaemia and infarction of the bowel supplied by the superior mesenteric artery.

Causes

Occlusive:

   Thombosis related to atheroma and other causes, e.g. blood dyscrasias, oral contraceptives

   Embolus from, e.g. myocardial infarct, atrial fibrillation, SBE

   Dissecting aneurysm

   Vasculitis

   Venous thrombosis — 5–10% cases

Non-occlusive:

   Reduction in perfusion as a result of myocardial infarct, cardiac failure, shock, hypotension, anoxia

Clinical features — Thrombosis related to atheroma usually occurs in the elderly who often have a history suggestive of mesenteric angina (see later). The other causes may be seen in younger patients *Early:*

periumbilical colic which is poorly localised, severe and persistent; *later*: vomiting and diarrhoea (which may be bloody). *Early*: no localising signs; *later*: fever, hypotension, tachycardia and signs of acute peritonitis.

Diagnosis — difficult in early stages but it should be thought of in a patient with severe pain and no abdominal signs who has history suggestive of mesenteric angina, signs of atheromatous disease elsewhere and/or disorder predisposing to arterial emboli. If suspected, the diagnosis can be confirmed by arteriography; however, often there is not enough time and diagnosis is made at laparotomy.

Investigations
1. WCC — neutrophil leucocytosis is the rule.
2. Plain abdominal X–ray normal early on but later, fluid levels and free gas.
3. Arteriography — vital if diagnosis is suspected and peritonitis has not yet developed.

Treatment
1. Resuscitation — vigorously with replacement of fluids, plasma and blood, oxygen, pressor agents (if indicated); treat associated diseases, if present
2. Surgery — urgent, as bowel will infarct if blood flow is not restored within six hours.
   a. If bowel is viable — remove thrombus or embolus and if necessary, revascularize gut with grafts, etc.
   b. If bowel viability is questionable — do as above but perform a 'second look' operation to check viability.
   c. If bowel is gangrenous — resect affected bowel. This may lead to an extensive small intestinal resection and can result in the short bowel syndrome, which may need special management.
3. Postoperative — heparin and antibiotics; intensive management on ITU with appropriate treatment for any complicating or associated disorders.

2. Chronic mesenteric ischaemia (Mesenteric angina)

An important diagnosis to make because eventually acute ischaemia and infarction occur.

Clinical features — usually seen in elderly arteriopaths with other disease, e.g. ischaemic heart disease, hypertension, diabetes.

Symptoms — epigastric colicky pain following 15 — 30 minutes after eating and lasting up to two hours (patients become afraid to eat), malabsorption and considerable weight loss.

Signs — weight loss, malnutrition, atheromatous disease elewhere, systolic bruit in upper abdomen

Investigations — Malabsorption (mild to moderate steatorrhoea is very common).

1. Arteriography — shows atheromatous and narrowed mesenteric arteries; significant narrowing (>50%) of two of the three major arteries is compatible with the diagnosis.
2. Ultrasound — may become important in the diagnosis of mesenteric vascular disease.

Diagnosis — should be suspected in elderly arteriopaths with a typical history who have compatible arteriographic features. Arteriography is *never* diagnostic.

Treatment

1. Medical — no value
2. Surgical — reconstruction of arteries and revascularization of bowel (not always possible); delay in surgery increases the chance of bowel infarction.

3. Ischaemic colitis

Ischaemia of the colon may be extensive or limited, severe or mild, reversible or irreversible. It most commonly affects 'watershed' areas between adjacent arterial supplies, e.g. splenic flexure, rectosigmoid area. Patients are usually elderly with atheroma, heart disease, diabetes or hypertension. In younger patients it may be associated with colonic disease, surgery, vasculitis, polycythaemia, shock, anoxia.

1. *Gangrenous ischaemic colitis* — irreversible colonic ischaemia with infarction; it is acute intestinal failure of bowel supplied by inferior mesenteric artery (see earlier for diagnosis and management); pain may start on left side of abdomen.
2. *Transient ischaemic colitis* — ischaemia, limited to colonic mucosa and submucosa.

Clinical features

Sudden onset colicky lower or left sided abdominal pain with nausea, vomiting and bloody diarrhoea; there may be a history of similar episodes previously.

Signs

Guarding and tenderness over the affected colon, fever, tachycardia, an abdominal mass or frank peritonitis.

Investigations

1. WCC — neutrophil leucocytosis
2. Sigmoidoscopy — normal in proximal disease; resembles non-specific proctitis in distal disease — histology of the rectal mucosa is similar.
3. Abdominal X-ray — may show the features of ischaemic colitis (see below) or of perforation.

4. Barium enema — typical features are narrowing, oedema, 'thumbprinting' and pseudopolyps at affected site.
5. Arteriography — not indicated.

Diagnosis

Diagnosis made on clinical features and barium enema appearance; extensive or distal disease may be difficult to distinguish from inflammatory bowel disease; clinical features may suggest acute diverticulitis.

Treatment

1. *Medical* — with symptomatic treatment, most cases settle in a few days; repeat enema after a week or so; in most cases, appearances return to normal but strictures may develop.
2. *Surgery* — only for deterioration with peritonitis; in last resort, surgery may be necessary for strictures.

INFECTIVE DIARRHOEA

General

Many organisms cause diarrhoea; clinical disorders vary from very mild and self-limiting to severe and life-threatening. The main clinical feature in most cases is diarrhoea possibly with associated fever, nausea, vomiting and abdominal colic. Blood, mucus and pus per rectum, tenesmus and systemic illness occur depending on the cause or severity of the infection. A full history is mandatory with particular reference to foreign travel, contacts (including sexual contacts), drug therapy (especially antibiotics). Full examination must include rectal examination, sigmoidoscopy, stool inspection.

Investigations

1. Sigmoidoscopy — to exclude colitis, ulceration, pseudomembranes.
2. Rectal swabs — remember special transport media for gonococci, etc.
3. Stool microscopy — for red cells, pus cells, organisms (including ova, cysts, parasites).
4. Stool culture.
5. Full blood count.
6. Viscosity or ESR; acute phase proteins.
7. Blood culture.
8. Serology — immmediately and in convalescent period.
9. Plain abdominal X-ray — to detect perforation, toxic dilatation and, in some cases, the extent of colonic inflammation.

Treatment

Be prepared to treat severe colonic infection in the same intensive way as in severe UC (see 'ulcerative colitis and Crohn's disease').

1. Replacement of fluid and electrolytes (especially potassium) i.v. in most cases, orally in mild cases.
2. Nil by mouth — if seriously ill; light diet — if mildly ill.
3. Symptomatic treatment — antidiarrhoeal agents, e.g. codeine phosphate 60–120 mg/day or loperamide 4–16 mg/day; do not give them to patients with moderate to severe colonic inflammation e.g. bacillary dysentery, because of the risks of toxic dilatation.
4. Antibiotics — avoid unless *specifically* indicated; even if a bacterial pathogen is isolated, e.g. salmonella, antibiotic therapy may lead to prolonged excretion of the bacteria and to antibiotic resistance. Severe systemic illness and infection with severely pathogenic organisms, e.g. *Salmonella typhi*, are indications for antibiotics.
5. Hygiene — scrupulous care with disposal and cleaning of contaminated specimens, instruments, crockery, bedclothes, clothes, etc. In severe infections, e.g. typhoid fever, barrier nursing is necessary.
6. Follow up — until organisms have been eliminated from stool, blood, etc.; in certain infections, there can be a high relapse rate and carrier states can occur.

Food poisoning

Diarrhoea after eating contaminated food; three main types:
1. Bacterial toxin — e.g. *Staphylococcus aureus*, *Bacillus cereus* — onset 1–6 hours after ingestion.
2. Infection, e.g. Salmonella species, Shigella species, *Bacillus cereus* — onset 24–48 hours after ingestion.
3. Chemical toxins.

Investigation and treatment — see earlier; antibiotics rarely indicated.

Gastroenteritis

Usually a self limiting form of diarrhoea which may be:
1. Viral, e.g. Rotavirus, various parvoviruses.
2. Bacterial, e.g. *E. coli*, Salmonella species, Shigella species — often seen in travellers (so-called 'Travellers' diarrhoea').

Investigation and treatment — see earlier; antibiotics are rarely indicated in bacterial gastroenteritis.

Salmonellosis

Three clinical syndromes:
Gastroenteritis/food poisoning
Salmonella colitis
Typhoid fever

Typhoid fever

Caused by *S. typhi*

Clinical features

1–3 week incubation period followed by insidious onset of fever, headache, cough, constipation, abdominal discomfort, bradycardia. After one week, diarrhoea (pea soup stools) in approximately 20% of cases. In second week, rose pink macules, abdominal distension, hepatomegaly, splenomegaly with step-wise increase in fever. During third week, complications may occur, e.g. intestinal perforation, ileus or haemorrhage. Gradual recovery after third or fourth week. A carrier state may occur.

Diagnosis

This depends on isolation of *S. typhi* from blood (first week) or faeces, urine or rectal swabs (second and third week). Serology may be unhelpful, although a rising 'O' antibody titre in a febrile illness is suggestive.

Treatment

1. Barrier nursing in hospital.
2. General measures, i.e. fluid replacement, etc.
3. Antibiotics — chloramphenicol 50 mg/kg/day in divided doses for 12 days is probably the treatment of choice; co-trimoxazole or ampicillin are effective alternatives.
4. Treat complications as they arise; surgery may be necessary.
5. Watch for relapse — common two weeks or so after cessation of therapy.

Prevention

Heat killed vaccine — 0.5 ml s.c. followed by 1 ml s.c. four weeks later; then booster dose 0.5 ml s.c.

Paratyphoid fever

Caused by *Salmonella paratyphi* A, B or C; milder than typhoid fever with a shorter incubation period; diagnosis and treatment similar to typhoid fever.

Shigellosis

Bacillary dysentery is caused by Shigella species of which there are 4 major strains, *S. dysenteriae*, *S. flexneri*, *S. boydii*, *S. sonnei* with numerous different serotypes.

Clinical features

This disease is a colitis varying from mild to severe; classic symptoms are fever, colicky abdominal pain and watery diarrhoea followed in 3–5 days by rectal burning, tenesmus and small volume bloody stools with mucus. Many cases (e.g. sonnei) are much milder with abdominal pain and diarrhoea. Bacteraemia is rare. Complications are intestinal perforation, toxic megacolon, reactive arthropathy. A chronic carrier state is rare.

Length of illness varies from a few days to several weeks. Sigmoidoscopy is very painful and shows a colitis.

Diagnosis
Isolation of a Shigella strain from stools. Other bacteria can cause the dysentery syndrome, e.g. Salmonella species, *Campylobacter fetus*, *Yersinia enterocolitica*.

Treatment
1. General measures but antidiarrhoeals can precipitate toxic megacolon. N.B. Shigellosis is highly contagious.
2. Antibiotics — can prolong Shigella excretion, therefore are only used for severe cases; ampicillin (resistance can occur) or co-trimoxazole for five days are drugs of choice.

Campylobacter enterocolitis

Commonest cause is *C. fetus* subspecies fetus; reservoir for infection is infected cattle, sheep, poultry, so usual mode of human infection is contaminated foods.

Clinical features
Incubation period of 1–3 days, then a coryzal prodromal illness followed by dysentery; diarrhoea may be bloody and biphasic. The illness lasts about a week but relapse is common. Minor infections may be asymptomatic.

Diagnosis — stool culture.

Treatment
1. General measures.
2. Erythromycin 500 mg qds for one week.

Yersiniosis

Two syndromes
1. Acute ileitis (usually caused by *Y. pseudotuberculosis*) — may mimic acute appendicitis or Crohn's disease clinically and Crohn's disease radiologically or at laparotomy.
2. Enteritis (usually caused by *Y. enterocolitica*) — similar to Salmonella or Shigella infections with small and large bowel inflammation.

Complications
Septicaemia, erythema nodosum, reactive arthropathy (Reiter's disease).

Diagnosis
Confirmed by isolation of organism from a lymph node or by rising antibody titres.

Treatment
Infection is usually self limiting and X-rays return to normal.
1. General measures.
2. Tetracycline or co-trimoxazole for severe cases only.

Clostridium difficile colitis (antibiotic associated colitis)

C. difficile and/or its toxin are frequently isolated from patients who have diarrhoea while taking antibiotics — particularly clindamycin, lincomycin and ampicillin. Antibiotic associated colitis is commoner in the elderly and in those with multiple antibiotic regimes.

Pseudomembranous colitis typically occurs but the disease may be much milder without obvious colonic pseudomembranes. *N.B.* there are other causes of pseudomembranous colitis, e.g. ischaemia, shock, surgery, other infections, inflammatory bowel disease.

Clinical features

Mild or very severe life threatening diarrhoea with mucus and occasionally frank blood PR. Any part of the colon may be affected, but the recto–sigmoid area is most commonly involved.

Investigations

As before; sigmoidoscopy may show normal mucosa, mild proctitis, severe ulcerative proctitis and/or frank pseudomembrane formation; the mucosa may be hidden by mucus. Faeces may be full of neutrophils. Barium enema appearances are non specific but show the affected areas.

Diagnosis

Diagnosis rests on finding *C. difficile* and/or its toxin in stool; there is usually (but not always) a history of recent antibiotic ingestion; pseudomembranes are not invariable; the main differential diagnosis is from other colonic infection and inflammatory bowel disease.

Treatment

1. General measures; avoid antidiarrhoeals because of the risk of toxic megacolon.
2. Vancomycin 1–2 g/day (in divided doses) or metronidazole 400 mg tds for one week.
3. Prednisolone — for very severe cases
4. Follow up — check stools for *C. difficile* and toxin; relapse is common requiring further courses of vancomycin or metronidazole.

Giardiasis

Caused by the protozoon, *Giardia lamblia*, which is the commonest gut parasite; particularly common in travellers from tropics and subtropics, but can be acquired in Europe especially in Leningrad. It may be seen in patients with immunoglobulin deficiency and in homosexuals.

Clinical features

Mild or severe; persistent or intermittent diarrhoea; features of malabsorption may occur as organism has a predilection for the proximal small bowel.

Investigations
As for other infective diarrhoeas; malabsorption investigation (see Ch. 10) may be necessary and steatorrhoea, malabsorption pattern on barium follow through and jejunal villous abnormalities may be found; after diagnosis exclude immunoglobulin deficiency.

Diagnosis
Stool microscopy reveals cysts in 50–80% cases but microscopy of jejunal juice aspirate is more accurate. On jejunal biopsy, trophozoites may be seen with difficulty on H and E staining. The most accurate way of showing the trophozoites and making the diagnosis is to wipe the jejunal mucosa on a slide and stain with Geimsa stain.

Treatment
Metronidazole 400 mg tds for one week or 2 g daily for three days; alternative is mepacrine 100 mg tds for one week; repeat courses may be required, if one course does not eliminate the organism.

Amoebic dysentery

Caused by protozoon *Entamoeba histolytica*; is widely distributed in tropics and subtropics; infection indicated by luminal cysts which cause few or no symptoms (carrier state) or trophozoites which invade the bowel mucosa; factors predisposing to invasion are largely unknown; there is a diffuse or patchy colitis particularly affecting the rectum, caecum and flexures.

Clinical features
Acute or insidious onset of diarrhoea, which may be bloody; tenesmus is absent; colonic tenderness and hepatomegaly (even without associated hepatic abscess) occur; severity is variable.

Complications
Hepatic abscess, intestinal perforation, toxic megacolon.

Investigations
As for other infectious diarrhoeas; sigmoidoscopy shows punched out ulcers with normal intervening mucosa or a diffuse proctocolitis.

Diagnosis
1. Microscopy — Amoebae may be seen in 'hot' stools, on rectal biopsy or in ulcer scrapings.
2. Serology — gel diffusion precipitation test is positive in invasive disease; the serological tests are useful for epidemiological studies only. *N.B.* severe amoebic dysentery can be difficult to differentiate clinically from severe UC and severe bacillary dysentery.

Treatment
1. General measures — avoid antidiarrhoeals because of the risks of toxic dilatation.
2. Antiamoebal therapy — Metronidazole 500 mg tds for 10 days; alternative is tinidazole (2 g daily for three days);

second line drugs are diloxanide furoate (500 mg tds) or tetracycline (250 mg qds) for 10 days, which are given for metronidazole resistance, and in all severe cases concurrently with metronidazole. Relapses requiring further treatment are common; carriers are treated with diloxanide furoate. Hepatic abscesses usually resolve with standard antiamoebal therapy but surgical drainage or wide-bore needle aspiration may be needed for large superficial abscesses.

Rectal gonorrhoea

Rectum is invaded by *Neisseria gonorrhoeae* as a result of anal intercourse and/or spread from the vagina.

Clinical features
Patients are asymptomatic or have diarrhoea, rectal burning, anal pruritus, tenesmus with pus, blood and/or mucus PR. Condylomata acuminata or anal fissures may coexist.

Investigation
As for other infectious diarrhoeas; proctosigmoidoscopy shows that inflammation rarely extends into the sigmoid colon.

Diagnosis
Proctoscopy shows a non specific proctitis with erythema and a mucopurulent exudate, therefore isolation of the organism from a culture is vital; adherent mucus should be swabbed via the proctoscope, avoiding faecal contamination, and the swab immediately transferred to a specific transport medium, e.g. Thayer–Martin plate. Rectal biopsy is usually unhelpful but may reveal gonoccoci. Other potential sites for gonococci, i.e. throat, cervix, urethra should be swabbed.

Treatment
Procaine penicillin 2–4 g im for 3 days preceded 30 min before each injection by probenecid, 1 g orally; this also eliminates pharyngeal gonorrhoea and any associated syphilis; ampicillin is an alternative; spectinomycin is indicated in penicillin sensitive patients or in treatment failures; relapse and/or reinfection is common.

Sexually related intestinal disease

An increasingly common problem, which is not confined to homosexuals, therefore 'gay bowel syndrome' is a misnomer. Sexually transmitted intestinal infections include gonorrhoea, giardiasis, amoebiasis, shigellosis, salmonellosis, campylobacter infections, syphilis, chlamydial infections and virus diseases, e.g. Herpes simplex.

CONSTIPATION

Investigation
See Ch 5.

Treatment
Constipation is not a disease but a symptom so treatment depends on its cause. However, general principles are:
1. *Treat underlying cause* e.g. perianal disorders, hypothyroidism, depression.
2. *General measures*:
   a. Education about colon function
   b. Encouragement of regular meals, regular defaecation attempts and regular exercise.
3. *Diet* — encourage a high fibre intake unless contraindicated by obstruction.
4. *Laxatives* — see later
5. *Other measures*, e.g. enemas, rectal washouts, colonic irrigation etc. Manual evacuation under anaesthetic may be necessary for severe cases especially if there is faecal impaction in the rectum or if the colon has to be cleared for barium enema, colonoscopy or surgery. Inorganic salt enemas, e.g. sodium phosphate, are useful in many cases and can be repeated as necessary. Rectal washouts and colonic irrigation with warm saline can be used for more resistant cases. Faecal impaction may require daily olive oil or dioctyl sodium sulphosuccinate enemas to soften the stool followed by saline washouts of the rectum and colon. Soap enemas are irritant and should never be used.
6. *Surgery* — indicated for Hirschsprung's disease or obstructing lesions. Colectomy and ileorectal anastomosis may be indicated for some cases of acquired megacolon and colonic inertia. Colostomy may be necessary for patients with severe colorectal dysfunction secondary to neurological disease or trauma.

Laxatives

The mode of action of most laxatives is not well understood and much that is written on the subject is probably incorrect. For convenience, laxatives can be classified into three broad groups:
1. *Bulk laxatives* — increase faecal weight and lower stool viscosity by increasing stool water.
   a. Hydrophilic agents, i.e. cellulose, mucilagenous seeds and gums (e.g. agar, Normacol, Isogel) and bran.

   b. Inorganic salts — soluble phosphates, tartrates and
      sulphates of sodium, potassium or magnesium.
      Magnesium sulphate is widely used.
 2. *Faecal softeners* — mode of action is uncertain.
    a. Dioctyl sodium sulphosuccinate (docusate sodium).
    b. Liquid paraffin.
 3. *Stimulant laxatives* — act directly on myenteric plexuses.
    a. Anthracine derivatives, e.g. senna, danthron, cascara.
    b. Phenylmethane derivatives, e.g. phenolphthalein,
       bisacodyl, sodium picosulphate, oxyphenisatin.
 4. *Other laxatives*
    a. Lactulose — colonic bacteria hydrolyse this synthetic
       disaccharide to short chain fatty acids which increase stool
       water by osmotic effects or by promoting colonic
       secretion.
    b. Castor oil — this hydroxylated long chain fatty acid
       (ricinoleic acid) is a powerful small and large intestinal
       secretagogue.

General principles of laxative use
 1. Use only when a diagnosis has been made; do not use if
    bowel obstruction is present (or suspected).
 2. Only use when absolutely necessary.
 3. Never use longer than is absolutely necessary. A lot of
    encouragement may be necessary to persuade a patient to
    discontinue laxative therapy.
 4. If laxatives are necessary long term, monitor regularly.
 5. Discourage the use of proprietary laxatives.
 6. For severe constipation, a stimulant laxative (e.g. senna) may
    be needed to initiate regular defaecation but change to
    gentler laxative when possible.
 7. If faecal impaction is present, clear rectum with enemas or
    washouts before starting laxative (usually a stimulant) by
    mouth.
 8. *Which laxative?*
    a. *First choice* — hydrophilic agent, e.g. Isogel 5–10 ml bd
       after meals, or at night; can cause flatulence and, if a
       stenosing lesion is present, blockage.
    b. *Second choice* — Lactulose, 15–30 ml daily; can cause
       diarrhoea and flatulence therefore adjust dose as
       necessary; may be combined with a hydrophilic agent.
    c. *Probable third choice* — dioctyl sodium sulphosuccinate,
       up to 500 mg daily in divided doses. *N.B.* It is often
       combined with a stimulant laxative in proprietary
       preparations — avoid these.
    d. *Use only if* **absolutely** *necessary*
       Anthracene laxatives, e.g. senna (2–4 tablets at night) can
       cause diarrhoea, colic, dehydration, hypokalaemia,

melanosis coli, cathartic colon; long term use leads to habituation.

Inorganic salts, e.g. magnesium sulphate; can cause diarrhoea, dehydration and electrolyte disorders.

e. **Never use**

Oxyphenisatin — causes liver damage.

Castor oil — causes severe water and electrolyte secretion

Liquid paraffin — inhalation causes lipoid pneumonia, absorption causes paraffinomas and anal seepage occurs causing pruritus.

Laxative abuse syndrome

Caused by long standing consumption of laxatives, especially stimulant laxatives. It can be easier to prevent than treat.

Two types:

1. Overt laxative abuse — patients with real or imagined long standing constipation who readily admit regular laxative ingestion.
2. Surreptitious laxative abuse — nearly always women with associated psychological problems such as anorexia nervosa; patients present with side effects of laxative ingestion without revealing or admitting to laxative ingestion. These patients sometimes abuse diuretics taken for imagined oedema.

Clinical features

Diarrhoea (often severe, especially in the surreptitious group), abdominal discomfort and bloating, tiredness, lethargy. Patients may present with complications such as dehydration, hypokalaemia, or hypokalaemic nephropathy.

Investigation and diagnosis

Diagnosis is not difficult in overt laxative takers but it can be very difficult in surreptitious abusers. The diagnosis should be considered in all patients with chronic diarrhoea that defies easy diagnosis, especially if the diarrhoea is osmotic in type and hypokalaemia is present.

1. Sigmoidoscopy and rectal biopsy — diagnosis is suggested by presence of melanosis coli macroscopically or on biopsy; is seen with anthracene laxative abuse and is reversible when laxative ingestion ceases.

2. Barium enema — is abnormal in 10% of surreptitious abusers because the cathartic colon is featureless, ahaustral and dilated, particularly on the right side; pseudostrictures are seen between dilated segments; histology shows damage to the myenteric plexus of the colon.

3. Serum electrolytes — hypokalaemia is common and can lead to hypokalaemic nephropathy; faecal sodium and water loss can cause secondary hyperaldosteronism.

4. Stool analysis — weight is usually greater than 250 g/day; electrolyte analysis and osmolality reveal an osmotic diarrhoea.

5. Anaemia, malabsorption with steatorrhoea, protein losing enteropathy, hypoglycaemia, glycosuria have been described.

6. Specific tests for laxatives:
   a. Urinary anthaquinolones — present in anthacene laxative ingestion.
   b. Alkalinization of stool and urine with sodium bicarbonate — goes pink if phenolphthalein is present.
   c. Faecal magnesium — elevated if magnesium salts have been ingested.
   d. Locker search while patient is otherwise engaged; this is vital in the investigation but is legally suspect.

Treatment — difficult

Overt abusers — education, treatment of constipation by dietary changes and introduction of gentler laxatives (see earlier), treatment of underlying causes of the constipation; weaning patients off laxatives can be very difficult.

Surreptitious abusers — confrontation with the diagnosis can lead to the patient going elsewhere with repetition of tests and may cause suicide. Patients should be given a chance to admit to laxative abuse. If she does not take the chance, regular follow up is necessary, treating symptoms and complications (especially hypokalaemia) as required. Psychiatric treatment should be offered for additional problems but is often unhelpful for the laxative abuser.

Cathartic colon — Colectomy may be necessary, if the colon fails to function after withdrawal of laxatives.

IRRITABLE BOWEL SYNDROME

The most common outpatient GI disorder in Britain.

Symptoms
Disturbance of bowel habit with diarrhoea and/or constipation, passage of mucus PR, abdominal pain (any site) and occasionally dyspepsia and nausea. Some patients have painless diarrhoea only.

Signs
Often none but tenderness over the colon, palpable spastic colon and colonic faecal masses may be found.

Investigations
To exclude other GI diseases (especially carcinoma and inflammatory bowel disease), the minimal investigations are:

1. Rectal examination, faecal occult blood testing and sigmoidoscopy.
2. Full blood count, acute phase proteins.
3. Serum proteins and serum iron.
4. Barium enema.

Diagnosis — by exclusion.

Management

1. Reassurance and explanation
2. High fibre diet
3. Drugs
   a. For pain — antispasmodics e.g. clinidium, mebeverine.
   b. For anxiety — a benzodiazepine.
   c. For constipation — lactulose or stool bulking agent, e.g. Isogel, Normacol.
   d. For diarrhoea — stool bulking agent or in the last resort, antidiarrhoeal agent, e.g. codeine phosphate.
4. Psychotherapy — hypnosis has been effective.
5. Antidepressants — may be indicated in a few cases, who are clinically depressed.

DIVERTICULAR DISEASE OF THE COLON

This is commonly found in later life and it is important to realise that many patients with diverticulosis do *not* have symptoms. It is important to be absolutely sure that the symptoms and signs *are* the result of diverticulosis and not some other, perhaps less obvious, disease.

Symptoms
Often none; if present, are similar to those of the irritable bowel syndrome (see above). Diverticulitis causes localised pain, diarrhoea and fever. Diverticular disease may present with one of its complications.

Signs
Often none; localised tenderness or mass over the colon; features of perforation or obstruction may be present.

Complications
Stricture, fistula, abscess, bleeding, perforation.

Investigations
Same as in irritable bowel syndrome (see above). If patient is ill and febrile, check blood and stool cultures and do plain abdominal X-ray rather than a barium enema which can be done when the acute diverticulitis has settled.

Diagnosis
Barium enema with compatible symptoms; acute diverticulitis is mainly a

clinical diagnosis; beware of ascribing lower GI tract bleeding to diverticular disease — look for other causes, e.g. carcinoma.

Treatment

1. Diverticular disease — same as irritable bowel syndrome (see above).
2. Diverticulitis — broad spectrum antibiotics, analgesics, i.v. fluid (for severe cases); if acute abdomen is present, consider laparotomy.
3. Complications — most require surgery.

COLORECTAL CARCINOMA

Deaths approximately 16 500/year (England and Wales); second most common carcinoma (after bronchus) making up about 16% of all malignant deaths; its prevalence is increasing; peak 55–60 years but 3% of cases are seen in patients less than 35 years of age; M : F ratio is 1 : 1.

Risk factors

These are largely unknown, but there is an increased prevalence of colorectal carcinoma in:

1. Benign adenoma (especially villous type).
2. Ulcerative colitis and Crohn's colitis.
3. Familial polyposis coli.
4. Gardner's syndrome (variant of polyposis coli with osteomas and soft tissue tumours).

Other risk factors may include diets high in fat and animal proteins or low in fibre. It is commoner in first degree relatives of patients with colorectal carcinoma.

Sites

In order of frequency — rectum, sigmoid colon, descending colon, caecum, ascending colon, transverse colon, flexures. 70% are in the rectum or colon within the pelvis; 3% are synchronous; 2% metachronous.

Pathology

1. Macroscopic — ulcerating (65%), fungating or polypoid (25%), colloid (10%), scirrhous. 'Benign' polyps may have foci of invasive carcinoma.
2. Microscopic — adenocarcinoma (95%), anaplastic (5%).

Symptoms

GI bleed (overt or occult), abdominal pain, change in bowel habit, nausea, vomiting, constitutional symptoms (anorexia, weight loss, malaise). Haemorrhoids can be a presenting feature (therefore rectal examination is obligatory in all new cases).

Rectal bleeding and constipation are common in left sided (especially rectal) carcinomas; iron deficiency anaemia, constitutional symptoms, nausea, vomiting are commoner in right sided lesions. Colorectal carcinomas may present with acute complications or with metastases. Caecal carcinoma may mimic acute appendicitis.

Signs

Anaemia, abdominal tenderness, signs of local complications or metastases, lesion and/or blood on rectal examination.

Metastases

Adjacent organs, local and regional lymph nodes, peritoneal cavity, liver, lungs, bone, brain. Tumours are staged by modified Dukes' classification:

        A. Tumour confined to bowel wall; no metastases — 15% of cases
        B. Tumour penetrating wall; no metastases — 35% of cases
        C. Regional lymph node metastases ⎫ 50% of cases
        D. Distant metastases ⎭

Complications

Obstruction, free perforation, local abscess, fistula.

Investigations and diagnosis

    1. Faecal occult blood.
    2. Sigmoidoscopy and biopsy — 55% of carcinomas are within reach of the 25 cm sigmoidoscope.
    3. Barium enema — double contrast.
    4. Colonoscopy — allows biopsy and brush cytology of radiologically suspect lesions, exclusion of synchronous carcinomas and assessment of polyps.
    5. Further assessment
        a. Full blood count
        b. Liver function tests
        c. Serum calcium
        d. Serum carcinoembryonic antigen
        e. Liver scan
        f. Bone scan

Treatment

    1. *Surgery* — the main principle is that the tumour is resected whether or not metastases are present, to prevent obstruction, tenesmus, bleeding, etc. Type of excision depends on the site and number of tumours and whether an underlying disease, e.g. ulcerative colitis is present. Cold resections are one stage procedures whereas obstruction or perforation may require a staged procedure with a temporary

colostomy. Second operation for recurrence or excision of
solitary hepatic metastasis may be indicated.
2. *Radiotherapy* — may be useful in treatment of recurrence,
metastases or as palliation; routine preoperative or post
operative radiotherapy is not indicated.
3. *Chemotherapy* — 5–fluorouracil may be useful in the
management of unresectable tumours and metastases.

Follow-up

Follow-up must be carried out after surgery because recurrence may be
successfully treated by further surgery. Indications of recurrence:
1. Symptoms — weight loss, GI bleeding, change in bowel
habit, abdominal pain (NB the last two may result from
adhesions).
2. Signs — abdominal mass, lymphadenopathy, hepatomegaly.
3. Investigations — raised ESR or serum alkaline phosphatase
or rising serum CEA; tumour on sigmoidoscopy, barium enema
or colonoscopy; metastases on chest X-ray, liver scan etc.
Colonoscopy is most useful test for recurrence and should be
done routinely at one year post operatively and thereafter at
2–3 year intervals.

Prognosis

This depends on grade of carcinoma and its spread (as assessed by
Dukes' grading). Overall five year survival is about 20% but only in 50%
can curative surgery be attempted. Of all operated patients, five year
survival is 45%; when broken down to Dukes' grades:
A — 80% 5 year survival
B — 60% 5 year survival
C — 30% 5 year survival
D — 5% 5 year survival

Screening

This is mandatory for all patients with familial polyposis coli, for patients
from families with a high incidence of colorectal carcinoma and for
patients with long standing ulcerative or Crohn's colitis. Role of
screening in average risk patients is not clear.
Therefore:
1. Patients from polyposis coli families — annual sigmoidoscopy
from age 10.
2. Patients from 'cancer' families — annual faecal occult blood
test and sigmoidoscopy every 3–5 years.
3. Ulcerative and Crohn's colitis — annual colonoscopy with
multiple biopsies in patients with total colitis for 7–10 years
or left sided colitis for 15–20 tears.
4. Average risk patients — yearly faecal occult blood over the
age 40–50 with sigmoidoscopy every 3–5 years.

BENIGN INTESTINAL POLYPS

Can be classified into:

        Neoplastic — adenoma, familial polyposis coli.
        Hamartomatous — juvenile polyp, Peutz-Jeghers syndrome.
        Inflammatory — benign lymphoid polyp, pseudopolyps in colitis.
        Unclassified — metaplastic (hyperplastic) polyp.

Neoplastic polyps (adenomas)

These are important because of their malignant potential.

Site

Frequently multiple; 77% are between splenic flexure and rectum; 48% are in the sigmoid colon.

Classification

Three types — tubular adenoma (75%), tubulovillous (intermediate) adenoma (10%), villous adenoma (15%).

Cancer risk

Greatest in villous adenoma, in polyps greater than 2 cm in diameter and in polyps with severe atypia (dysplasia). 46% of large (> 2 cm) adenomas are malignant and 60% of large adenomas, are of villous type. 5% of tubular adenomas, 23% of intermediate adenomas and 41% of villous adenomas are malignant. With severe atypia in tubular adenoma, there is a 1 in 4 risk of cancer.

Clinical

Rare below 30 years of age; progressively more common with age. Frequently symptomless but can cause pain, GI bleeding, change in bowel habit. Large villous adenomas can cause watery diarrhoea, mucus PR and hypokalaemia. Rectal examination may reveal polyp but a sessile villous adenoma may be so soft that it is missed.

Investigation and diagnosis

    1. Sigmoidoscopy — 50% of polyps are within reach of the 25 cm sigmoidoscope.
    2. Barium enema — must be double contrast.
    3. Colonoscopy — allows inspection, biopsy, brush cytology and removal of polyps. All polyps greater than 1 cm in diameter should be examined colonoscopically. If polyps are present on sigmoidoscopy but barium enema is normal, colonoscopy is indicated.

Treatment

Treatment should be considered for all polyps greater than 1 cm in diameter.

    1. Low rectal polyps — if pedunculated, removal with diathermy snare via flexible sigmoidoscopy; if sessile, electrofulguration.

2. Colonic or high rectal polyps — if pedunculated, colonoscopic (or flexible sigmoidoscopic) polypectomy with diathermy snare; if sessile, surgical polypectomy via colotomy should be considered especially if atypia is present. The whole polyp must be sent for histology; if a focus of invasive carcinoma is present but the excision line is clear, no immediate action is necessary but repeat colonoscopy in a few months; if excision line is invaded, colectomy is indicated.

Follow up
Check colonoscopy every two years

Familial Polyposis Coli

Autosomal dominant disorder with incomplete penetrance so only 40% of children at risk are affected. Multiple adenomatous polyps are present in the large bowel and the rectum is *always* affected. Polyps usually appear after 10 years of age, symptoms usually appear after 30 years of age and malignancy usually appears in the late thirties. 50% of cases will develop carcinoma.

Symptoms
Abdominal pain, diarrhoea, GI bleeding, mucus PR. Two-thirds have a carcinoma at presentation.

Diagnosis
Sigmoidoscopy and biopsy.
Barium enema — double contrast.

Treatment
Total colectomy with ileo–rectal anastomosis and electrofulguration of rectal polyps. If rectal carcinoma is present at diagnosis — panproctocolectomy.

Follow-up
Follow-up in those with an ileorectal anastomosis, proctoscopy and repeat fulguration at regular intervals (initially three months) for life.

Screening relatives
All first degree relatives should be offered yearly sigmoidoscopy from the age of 10, or as soon as possible after that age.

11. PANCREATIC DISEASE

ACUTE PANCREATITIS

Predisposing causes

        gallstones
        alcohol
        hypercalcaemia
        hyperlipidaemia
        trauma
        ERCP examination
        infection, e.g. mumps
        drugs, e.g. corticosteroids, thiazides, azathioprine
        hereditary pancreatitis

Symptoms

Sudden onset acute abdominal pain (typically severe, epigastric, boring through to back), vomiting, abdominal distension

Signs

Hypotension. Temperature initially low associated with shock but pyrexia develops after few hours. Abdomen rigid, motionless, with signs of peritonism. As ileus develops, bowel sounds lost and moderate distension occurs. Epigastric mass may develop with pseudocyst or abscess formation. Ascites not unusual in severe cases. Staining in flanks or periumbilical regions rare except in severe cases (Grey–Turner's and Cullen's signs). Slight to moderate jaundice often develops. Pulmonary complications and renal failure may be manifest as dyspnoea, cyanosis and oliguria.

Some patients with quite severe acute pancreatitis may exhibit surprisingly few signs and occasional patients may be more or less symptom free.

Other complications — haemorrhage, thrombophlebitis, fat necrosis, secondary infection.

Diagnosis

In most patients the diagnosis is easy with typical clinical picture and large rise in serum amylase level (>1000 Somogyi u). Confusion can occur with some other intra-abdominal pathologies, which can also cause large increases in serum amylase levels — e.g. afferent loop obstruction after polya gastrectomy, occasional cases of pelvic inflammatory disease and perforated peptic ulcer. More commonly, diagnostic difficulties arise because of normal serum amylase levels in the presence of true pancreatitis. In this situation, renal clearance of amylase exceeds production rate. Diagnosis can then be achieved by measurement of urinary amylase level.

Investigations

1. Serum and urinary amylase levels; in difficult cases aspirate peritoneal cavity for fluid — if present, measure amylase content; act similarly if pleural effusions are present.
2. Take blood for:
   a Crossmatching.
   b. Several blood cultures.
   c. Full blood count — neutrophil leucocytosis and anaemia are common.
   d. Urea, electrolytes, and plasma proteins to assess degree of hydration and baseline renal function.
   e. Serum calcium and magnesium estimations.
   f. Blood sugar — transient elevation may occur.
   g. Methaemalbumin — present in serum in haemorrhagic pancreatitis which has a much higher mortality.
3. Plain films of abdomen and chest
   a. Calcified gallstones may have an aetiological significance.
   b. Pleural effusions and 'pneumonic' changes (usually left-sided) indicate severe disease.
   c. Look for evidence of perforated abdominal viscus or other pathology.
4. Commence fluid balance charts and monitor urinary output carefully.
5. Ultrasound examination of biliary tree as soon as possible. Oedema and haemorrhage may later obscure the ultrasound diagnosis of biliary tract stones.
6. Serum for virology titres (mumps, etc.)

Management

1. Initial mortality is high in untreated cases and is caused by shock. All cases should have a CVP line and an intravenous line placed early.
2. Pass nasogastric tube for continuous gastric aspiration — this is mainly to treat the accompanying ileus rather than to decrease pancreatic stimulation.
3. Analgesia — e.g. pethidine 50–100 mg i.m., if pain despite gastric suction.

4. Ensure good hydration with intravenous saline once CVP has been restored with plasma to ensure adequate circulating blood volume and renal perfusion.
5. Ensure good oxygenation to minimise the development of 'shock lung' — commonly misdiagnosed as pneumonia in this situation.
6. Hypocalcaemia (and hypomagnesaemia) occur in severe cases and should be corrected intravenously. ECG monitoring is helpful.
7. Consider the need for surgical treatment:
   a. *Gallstones*
      Biliary tract stones, especially common duct stones should probably be removed surgically or at endoscopic sphincterotomy. The evidence indicates that this procedure can be performed without increasing disease mortality. Operations on the pancreas itself are controversial. There is no clear evidence that operating on the pancreas in the absence of complications benefits the course of the disease.
   b. *Complications*
      Monitor abdominal signs including girth. Repeat abdominal ultrasound to detect:
      Abscess — usually requires surgical drainage
      Pseudocyst — often requires surgical drainage unless small and non-progressive
   c. *Progressive deterioration* — especially if diagnosis is in doubt
8. Haemodialysis — may be required for progressive renal failure
9. Controversial treatment — atropine or glucagon to decrease pancreatic secretion, peritoneal lavage, antibiotics.

CHRONIC PANCREATITIS

Causes

Alcohol (most important)
Gallstones
Hyperparathyroidism
Malnutrition
Hereditary pancreatitis
Trauma

Clinical features

Pain — epigastric, radiating to back, worse on eating or drinking alcohol.
Weight loss due to:
1. Recent onset diabetes mellitus.

2. Steatorrhoea — can be gross.
3. Anorexia — especially in the alcoholic.

Signs are usually unimpressive.

Complications

Pancreatic pseudocyst, pancreatic ascites, obstructive jaundice.

Diagnosis

Can be difficult in the early stages. Sometimes difficult to differentiate from carcinoma.

Requires:

1. *Assessment of gross anatomy*
   a. Plain X-ray of abdomen for pancreatic calcification.
   b. Ultrasound of pancreas.
   c. Endoscopic retrograde pancreatography (ERCP).
   d. Computerised X-ray tomography.
2. *Assessment of exocrine function*
   a. By tests requiring duodenal intubation (secretin/pancreozymin stimulation test, Lundh test) or by indirect tubeless test (fluorescein dilaurate test, n-benzoyl-n-tyrosyl-para-aminobenzoic acid test).

   Advanced disease is usually present before changes in exocrine function become apparent. Probably the most sensitive test for detecting relatively early exocrine changes is measurement of enzyme and bicarbonate output on maximal stimulation using secretin/cholecystokinin infusions.
   b. Faecal fat and faecal nitrogen — increased
3. *Assessment of endocrine function* — fasting blood glucose, glucose tolerance test, glycosylated haemoglobin levels.

N.B. Any or all tests may remain normal even in the presence of histologically proven chronic pancreatitis.

Investigations

Preceded by careful history with respect to alcohol ingestion.

1. Blood tests
   a. Amylase — may be elevated in co-existent acute inflammation or pseudocyst formation.
   b. Liver function tests — mild elevation of bilirubin, alkaline phosphatase and transaminases are common especially in alcoholics; gross elevations of bilirubin and alkaline phosphatase in obstructive jaundice; serum albumin is usually well preserved.
   c. Check for aetiological factors, e.g. alcohol (MCV serum γ GT and ethanol) lipids, calcium.

    d. Blood sugar.

    e. Vitamins A,D,K, folic acid, B_{12}.

2. Faeces — fat and nitrogen contents are elevated in gross exocrine failure; stool microscopy may show fat globules and undigested meat fibres.

3. Consider co-existing multisystem disease due to alcohol abuse, e.g. neuropathy, cardiomyopathy, and investigate if indicated.

4. Visualize the biliary tree — by ultrasound, for evidence of extrahepatic obstruction and calculi, and cholangiography (ERCP) for strictures, etc.

5. Visualize the pancreatic duct by endoscopic retrograde pancreatography.

Management

1. Correct all nutritional deficiencies — especially if of alcoholic aetiology or if malabsorption is present.

2. Pain — a prominent and distressing feature but tends to resolve as pancreatic destruction becomes complete. Ensure abstinence from alcohol. Use non-narcotic analagesics whenever possible, but sublingual buprenorphine is very effective. Some patients respond to pancreatic enzyme replacement therapy by mouth even in the absence of overt exocrine insufficiency. Anticholinergics rarely helpful. For refractory pain consider:

    a. Transcutaneous nerve stimulator.

    b. Percutaneous coeliac plexus block.

    c. Pancreatic surgery in appropriate cases.

3. Malabsorption — usually responds to oral replacement of pancreatic enzymes, but remember:

    a. Replacement dose must be individually tailored and is usually large.

    b. Enzymes inactivated by heat and acid should not be sprinkled on hot foods and should be protected from low intragastric pH by large doses of liquid antacids or H_2 receptor antagonists.

    c. Low fat diet may also be necessary to relieve some symptoms, e.g. diarrhoea — start at 40 g fat/day and increase until symptoms develop.

4. Diabetes — treated as any other Type 1 diabetes with calorie restriction and insulin. Contrary to popular belief, diabetes secondary to pancreatic disease is not more difficult to treat.

5. Role of surgery — opinions on this vary. Co-existing biliary tract disease should be treated effectively and early. Indications for surgery on the pancreas itself are usually intractable pain, but results for pain relief can be

disappointing. Some patients with dilated pancreatic ducts can respond dramatically to surgical decompression.

Pancreatectomy is probably best avoided if:

a. Patient continues to drink alcohol.

b. The patient is not yet diabetic.

c. Exocrine function remains good.

Surgery is required for complications of pseudocyst, ascites and obstructive jaundice.

PANCREATIC CARCINOMA

Responsible for 5.5% of all deaths from cancer, being exceeded only by lung, colorectal and breast cancer and incidence is rising. 75% patients over 60 years at diagnosis. M:F ratio is 1.6:1.

Risk factors

Smoking

Diet — especially fat

Occupation — coke and chemical workers

Diabetes mellitus — especially in females

Gallstones

Chronic pancreatitis (possibly)

Pathology

1. Macroscopic — head (70%) usually obstructs pancreatic and biliary ducts; spreads to duodenum and local lymph nodes; body and tail (30%) spreads to superior mesenteric vessels, portal vein and colon.

2. Microscopic — adenocarcinoma: ductal type (80–90%), acinar type (10–20%). Other types include squamous cell, islet–cell and cystadenocarcinoma.

3. Metastases — in about 60% of cases, especially to liver, abdominal lymph nodes, peritoneum, lungs.

Symptoms

Weight loss, jaundice, abdominal pain, nausea, vomiting, change in bowel habit, dark urine, pale stools, pruritus.

Signs

Hepatomegaly, jaundice, abdominal mass, palpable gallbladder, thrombophlebitis, ascites.

Investigations and diagnosis

By the time symptoms develop and currently available investigations can confirm the diagnosis, pancreatic carcinoma is usually beyond the stage when surgical removal is possible.

1. Full blood count, ESR (elevated in nearly all cases).

2. Serum bilirubin alkaline phosphatase, amylase. An oral glucose tolerance test is abnormal in more than 50% of patients.
3. Exocrine pancreatic function tests may show reduced volume of secretion but normal bicarbonate concentration. Frequently the results are indistinguishable from those obtained in chronic pancreatitis.
4. Radiology — plain abdominal X-ray may show pancreatic calcification, an abdominal mass, or pancreatic abscess. Hypotonic duodenography may show tumour in head of pancreas.
5. Ultrasound — can detect tumours 2 cm or larger. Very observer dependent.
6. CT scan — can detect an abnormal pancreas in 80% cases.
7. Endoscopic retrograde cholangiopancreatography (ERCP) — most accurate test to distinguish between chronic pancreatitis and pancreatic cancer. Cannulation failure 15–20%. Specimens for cytology can be obtained. Cytology specimens may also be obtained pre-operatively by CT or ultrasound guided fine needle aspiration or intraoperatively by direct puncture.
8. Angiography — selective arteriography will delineate vascular anatomy prior to surgery — important in determining resectability.
9. Laparoscopy — enables pancreas to be visualised and histology/cytology specimens to be obtained. Laparotomy may be avoided, if advanced intra-abdominal disease is confirmed.
10. Laparotomy with pancreatic biopsy — obtained directly or transduodenally by needle biopsy, or by wedge biopsy. Haemorrhage, pancreatitis, fistula formation are complications.

Treatment

1. Surgery

  a. Laparotomy
  This is usually necessary to confirm the diagnosis except in cases of disseminated cancer. Biopsy is necessary to differentiate between chronic pancreatitis and carcinoma. Laparotomy can also help in identifying carcinomas of ampulla, duodenum and intrapancreatic common bile duct which have a much better prognosis after resection than carcinoma of head of pancreas.

  b. Resection
  Pancreaticoduodenectomy (Whipple's operation) is the

operation of choice for carcinoma of head of pancreas although multicentric tumours, tumour still present at line of resection, and leakage at pancreaticojejunal anastomosis are hazards. Because of this total pancreatectomy and splenectomy have been advocated. The operative mortality is no greater, but neither is the five year survival.

 c. *Palliation*

 Bypass operations to relieve obstructive jaundice and to prevent duodenal obstruction may need to be performed. Internal drainage of the biliary tree may be carried out at PTC or ERCP and tubes left in situ.

2. Radiotherapy

Has no part to play alone in treating irresectable tumours but in combination with chemotherapy there is some evidence of benefit.

3. Chemotherapy

5-Fluorouracil has been used most often. Response is poor. In combination with radiotherapy there may be some benefit.

4. Other measures

Severe pain is often a feature and attention to analgesia using morphine or other narcotic agents is important. Percutaneous coeliac axis block is also effective.

Prognosis

Extremely poor. Five year survival after resection of carcinoma in head is 5%. Average survival following a bypass procedure is four months compared to 17 months after resection. Resection is possible in only 12%.

12. HEPATIC DISEASE

ACUTE VIRAL HEPATITIS

Causes

> Hepatitis A (HAV)
> Hepatitis B (HBV)
> Non A, Non B
> Others — Epstein–Barr (infectious mononucleosis)
> > Cytomegalovirus
> > Herpes simplex
> > Coxsackie B
> > Adenovirus
> > Varicella
> > Yellow fever
> > Delta agent (only seen in HBsAg carriers)

The term hepatitis usually refers to HAV, HBV, or non A, non B infection.

N.B. Acute hepatocellular inflammation may also be caused by drugs and toxins.

Pathology

Viral hepatitis is a multisystem disease predominantly affecting the liver; this typically shows centrizonal necrosis.

Clinical features

Generally the same for all three types of viral hepatitis. A careful history is vital to note jaundiced contacts, sexual preference, recent travel, any injections or blood transfusions, drug history (iatrogenic or social), tatoos, ingestion of shell fish (can harbour HAV).

Typical attack — prodromal period of 3–4 days (can be as long as 2–3 weeks) with malaise, lethargy, anorexia, nausea, vomiting, loss of taste, loss of desire for cigarettes or alcohol, headache, mild pyrexia, or mild diarrhoea. Right upper quadrant discomfort and pain may occur. As prodromal symptoms settle and the patient feels better, urine darkens, stools become paler and jaundice appears. *Signs* — jaundice, smooth tender hepatomegaly. Splenomegaly occurs in 20% and transient spider naevi may be seen; do not miss stigmata of chronic liver disease if present.

Jaundice usually lasts 1–4 weeks, but fatigue and malaise may last several weeks (or even longer in the 'post-hepatitis syndrome'); blood tests are normal by 6 months. *Mild attacks* may be anicteric; HBV infection may be more severe with a prolonged illness and a prodromal serum sickness like illness with arthritis, urticaria, etc.

Relapses

May occur and are usually milder than the first attack (may be anicteric); may be multiple; recovery is usually complete but relapses may indicate progression to chronic liver disease.

Complications

Prolonged cholestasis, acute fulminant liver failure (very rare with HAV), chronic liver disease (not with HAV), bone marrow aplasia, myocarditis, acute pancreatitis, Coomb's positive haemolytic anaemia. Non hepatic complications do not occur with non A, non B hepatitis.

Investigations

1. Blood tests
   a. Full blood count — leucopenia (lymphopenia and/or neutropenia) may occur in prodromal period; atypical lymphoid cells may be seen (if present, exclude infectious mononucleosis with a Paul–Bunnell test).
   b. Coagulation screen (prothrombin time; platelet count; activated partial thromboplastin time) — mild prolongation of prothrombin time is common; severe derangement of clotting may indicate fulminant hepatitis.
   c. Liver function tests — bilirubin rises (height of bilirubin rise tends to correlate with the length of the clinical course); alkaline phosphatase rises at most to 3 times the upper limits of normal; serum transaminases rise indicating hepatocellular necrosis — the peak is 1–2 days before and after the onset of jaundice — rapid falls after very high levels may indicate impending fulminant hepatic failure; serum proteins are normal.
   d. Diagnosis of cause:
      (i) Hepatitis virus markers — see below
      (ii) Tests for other viral causes — necessary if hepatitis does not seem to be due to HAV, HBV or non A non B virus.
   e. Other tests — ESR is raised; serum IgM, IgG, iron and B_{12} may be raised; low titres of smooth muscle antibodies may be detected.
2. Urine tests
   a. Bilirubin — is detected in urine before jaundice appears, and disappears as cholestasis resolves.
   b. Urobilinogen appears in urine late in the pre-icteric phase, disappears when cholestasis is complete, reappears when cholestasis begins to recover and disappears when the patient recovers.

3. Liver biopsy — not necessary as routine, may be indicated in patients with atypical clinical features, with prolonged cholestasis, in those taking potentially hepatotoxic drugs and in those in whom an acute exacerbation of chronic liver disease cannot be excluded.

Diagnosis

Easy in most cases on clinical features and liver function tests; more difficult in anicteric hepatitis or in the prodromal phase (when elevation of serum transaminases will suggest diagnosis) and in the elderly or those presenting with prolonged cholestasis — liver biopsy may be necessary in these situations.

Hepatitis A (HAV)

It may occur sporadically or in epidemics; incubation period is 15–50 days; spread is normally by faeco–oral route — parenteral spread is rare.

Clinical features and prognosis

Commonest in children aged 5–15 years but can occur at any age; anicteric cases are common and are often diagnosed as gastroenteritis; the course is usually mild and mortality is very low (<1%) but fatal and fulminant cases can occur; chronicity does *not* occur.

Diagnosis

1. Identification of virus in stool — possible two weeks before and 1–2 weeks after the onset of jaundice — not used routinely.
2. HAV antibodies — anti HAV appears as HAV clears from stool, reaching a maximum several months after the attack and is detectable for years; a rising titre (seen in only 50% of cases) indicates infection. IgM anti–HAV lasts 2–6 months after attack and indicates recent infection.

Hepatitis B (HBV)

It is spread largely in blood and blood products but also in semen and saliva; transmission occurs parenterally or by sexual or intimate contact; incubation period is usually about 6 weeks but may be up to 6 months; carrier rate varies in different parts of the world (0.1–0.2% in USA and UK; 15% or more in parts of Africa and Far East).

Groups at special risk of having HBV

Drug addicts, male homosexuals, patients from the Mediterranean, Africa or Far East, patients and staff from mental subnormality hospitals, other hospital staff, babies of infected mothers, patients regularly receiving blood products (especially in countries where blood donors are paid).

Clinical features and prognosis

Subclinical attacks and reinfections may occur. The illness tends to be more severe than HAV infections. Features suggesting immune complex deposition may be present — e.g. serum sickness like syndrome, glomerulonephritis, polyarteritis.

Mortality is higher than in HAV or non A, non B infections and HBV is the commonest cause of fulminant viral hepatitis. About 10% of patients with acute HBV infection fail to clear the virus and become carriers. Chronic liver disease is associated with persisting HBV infection.

Diagnosis

1. *Hepatitis B markers*:
   a. Hepatitis B surface antigen (HBsAg) — appears in blood just before clinical symptoms develop and usually disappears by three months; persistence beyond six months suggests carrier status (but not necessarily infectivity).
   b. Antibody to HBsAg (anti-HBs) — appears in blood up to three months after illness and persists (indicating a previous HBV infection). Not every patient with HBV infection develops anti-HBs. Anti-HBs appears to confer immunity to HBV.
   c. Hepatitis B 'e' antigen (HBeAg) — this is probably part of the HBV core and appears in the blood after one week of illness and disappears in about two weeks; its presence indicates high infectivity and persistence implies carrier status. HBeAg can spontaneously convert to anti-HBe in carriers when the virus is incorporated into the liver cell DNA. This may be associated with a lobular hepatitis which may be mistaken for an exacerbation, re-infection or new virus infection — such as delta agent.
   d. Antibody to HBeAg (anti-HBe) — as HBeAg disappears from the blood, anti-HBe appears which lasts for many months.
   e. Antibody to Hepatitis B core antigen (anti-HBc) — appears as illness starts and can be useful if HBV is suspected as the cause of the hepatitis but HBsAg has cleared and anti-HBs is not yet positive.
   f. Other markers (e.g. HBcAg, DNA polymerase) are not indicated for routine clinical assessment.

2. *Virus identification*
   This is not indicated routinely, although HBsAg may be stained orange with orcein and seen in hepatocytes on liver biopsy as orcein bodies.

Non A, non B hepatitis

Epidemic pattern resembles HBV. It is largely spread by blood and blood products, accounting for 75% of post transfusion hepatitis. The virus (viruses) responsible have not been identified and any antibody response is weak. Incubation period is long (about 7 weeks) or short (1–4 weeks).

Clinical features and prognosis
Usually a mild illness, which is often subclinical or anicteric. Fulminant hepatitis can occur. Course may be prolonged and about 25% develop mild chronic hepatitis but chronic active hepatitis and cirrhosis may also develop.

Diagnosis
By exclusion of HAV, HBV and other viruses.

MANAGEMENT OF ACUTE VIRAL HEPATITIS

1. Treatment of acute attack — *N.B.* no treatment alters the course of the illness.
   a. Bed rest followed by a convalescent period, after patient feels well and liver tenderness and jaundice have resolved.
   b. Careful disposal of linen, excreta, crockery, etc.
   c. Diet — low fat high calorie is best tolerated during attack; high protein during convalescence.
   d. Corticosteroids — probably do not influence course of hepatitis but in patients with prolonged cholestasis, persisting jaundice, or raised serum globulins and transaminases, steroids improve liver function and the patient's symptoms. Relapse can occur when they are stopped and steroids may perpetuate HBV infection.
   e. Fulminant hepatitis — see later.
2. Follow-up — regularly until the liver function tests are normal and HBsAg has been cleared. If liver remains abnormal at six months, consider liver biopsy to assess progression to chronicity. Avoid alcohol for 12 months after acute attack.

PREVENTION

1. General public health measures — e.g. improved sanitation, education of the public, screening of blood donors, careful disposal of infected or potentially infected linen, crockery, foodstuffs, excreta, tissue and blood samples, surgical instruments, needles, etc.
2. HAV —
   a. Vaccination not available.
   b. Immune serum globulin — prevents or modifies HAV

infection if given within 1–2 weeks of exposure; not necessary if antibodies to HAV are present. Dose is 0.02 ml/kg i.m.; if risk is recurring (e.g. travel to high risk areas) 0.05 ml/kg i.m. every six months.

3. HBV —
   a. Vaccination — dose is 1 ml i.m. initially and repeated at one and six months; check anti-HBs response. Vaccination not necessary if patients have HBsAg or anti HBs in their serum.
   b. Hepatitis B immunoglobulin — after exposure it reduces the incidence but prolongs the incubation period of hepatitis. Dose is 5 ml i.m. within two days of exposure (e.g. needle stick) and repeat at about 28 days.
4. Non A, non B — no preventive treatment available.

ACUTE (FULMINANT) HEPATIC FAILURE

Causes

Viral hepatitis
Drugs, e.g. paracetamol, halothane
Toxins, e.g. *Amanita phalloides* (mushrooms)
Gram negative septicaemia
Fatty liver of pregnancy — very rare
N.B. Acute alcoholic hepatitis may present similarly

Clinical features

Usually a short history. Earliest features are frequently neuropsychiatric (see section on 'Hepatic encephalopathy' below) and may precede jaundice. However, acute fulminant hepatic failure may only appear when patient has become deeply jaundiced. Foetor is present, but flapping tremor may be transient. Neuropsychiatric features progress to coma, decerebrate rigidity, fits, respiratory and circulatory disorders and depression and death. The liver is usually small. It is vital to look for features of alcohol excess and chronic liver disease.

Investigations

1. Full blood count — neutrophil leucocytosis may be found.
2. Coagulation tests (prothrombin time, activated partial thromboplastin time) become grossly deranged and their severity is proportional to the outcome.
3. Blood for grouping and, if necessary, crossmatch.
4. Biochemistry:
   a. Serum urea and electrolytes.

    b. Urine electrolytes.

    c. Liver function tests — bilirubin steadily rises but is not a good prognostic guide; serum transaminases may be very low.

    d. Serum proteins — serum albumin may fall and this is a bad sign.

    e. Serum immunoglobulins.

    f. Urine aminoacids — aminoaciduria is usual.

    g. Blood sugar needs close monitoring as hypoglycaemia may be severe and sudden.

    h. Serum amylase — acute pancreatitis is a complication.

5. Search for infection:

    a. Hepatitis A and B markers

    b. Virological studies on faeces, blood, etc.

    c. Cultures of blood, urine, sputum etc. for bacteria.

6. ECG.

7. Chest X-ray.

8. EEG.

9. Other tests may be indicated, e.g. blood alcohol, blood drug or toxin levels, CSF examination (if other neurological disease cannot be excluded).

10. Liver biopsy — rarely possible because of deranged coagulation

Management

Aim is to provide intensive supportive care for the patient until such time as liver function returns.

    1. General measures

        a. Barrier nursing.

        b. IV line; CVP line.

        c. Indwelling urinary catheter.

        d. Nasogastric tube.

        e. Careful monitoring of fluid balance.

    2. Clinical assessment

        a. Temperature, pulse and BP at least hourly.

        b. Grade coma — two hourly (see later).

        c. Blood sugar every hour (by 'Dextrostix' or equivalent).

        d. Daily FBC, urea and electrolytes, prothrombin time.

        e. Examine for evidence of fluid retention daily.

    3. Treatment of problems

        a. Hepatic encephalopathy — no protein in diet, neomycin 1 g orally 4 hourly ± lactulose 10 ml qds, magnesium sulphate enema, no sedation (if possible). L-dopa may transiently arouse comatose patients.

        b. Cerebral oedema — steroids or mannitol are not helpful.

    c. Hypoglycaemia — is prevented by maintaining 10% glucose i.v. infusion (up to 3 l/24 h) and add 100–200 mmol potassium chloride daily (if urine output is satisfactory); treat hypoglycaemia with 100 ml 50% glucose i.v.

    d. Renal failure — haemodialysis may be needed.

    e. Respiratory failure — oxygen, intubation, ventilation.

    f. Circulatory failure — avoid volume depletion, monitor heart by ECG

    g. Infection — treat vigorously when there is a definite indication; do not give routine antibiotics.

    h. Bleeding — give vitamin K, whole blood, fresh frozen plasma, platelets as indicated; avoid arterial punctures; give maintenance H_2 blocker to reduce risk of gastric bleeding.

4. Corticosteroids
No evidence for benefit; may be harmful causing gastric erosions, acute pancreatitis, infection.

5. Artificial hepatic support and liver transplantation
Largely experimental but are available in a few centres.

Prognosis

Mortality is high and patients with long or deep coma or who are older do worse. If the patient survives, recovery is usually complete and chronic liver damage is rare.

CHRONIC HEPATITIS

This is chronic inflammation within the liver which has persisted without improvement for at least six months. There are three types:
    1. Chronic persistent hepatitis
    2. Chronic lobular hepatitis
    3. Chronic active hepatitis
Each type is defined on pathological criteria at liver biopsy.

Chronic persistent hepatitis

Causes
    HBV
    Non A, non B
    Unknown
    Similar histological appearances may be seen in patients after acute alcoholic hepatitis and in those with chronic inflammation (e.g. ulcerative colitis).

Clinical features
Commoner in males; may be no symptoms or mild malaise, lethargy, anorexia and right upper quadrant discomfort. *Signs* — none or mild liver tenderness; jaundice is rare and stigmata of chronic liver disease do not occur.

Investigations
1. Liver function tests — serum transaminases are usually raised and levels fluctuate. Serum bilirubin, alkaline phosphatase and globulins are normal or minimally raised.
2. HBV markers.
3. Liver biopsy — makes diagnosis; unhelpful within six months of an acute attack of viral hepatitis, as features may be the same as those of acute viral hepatitis.

Treatment
Reassurance; no specific therapy required.

Prognosis
In most cases excellent; progression to cirrhosis may occur with HBV and non A non B infection.

Chronic lobular hepatitis

Rare; cause is unknown or may follow non A, non B hepatitis; clinical features and investigations are similar to chronic persistent hepatitis but it tends to run a remitting and relapsing course; treatment is corticosteroids; prognosis is excellent but cirrhosis may develop.

Chronic active hepatitis

Causes

Autoimmune ('Lupoid' hepatitis)
HBV
Non A, non B
Cytomegalovirus (in children)
Drugs e.g. methyldopa, oxyphenisatin, isoniazid
α-1 antitrypsin deficiency
Alcohol
Wilson's disease

Autoimmune (HBsAg negative) chronic active hepatitis
This is seen in young adults and 75% of cases are in females.

Symptoms — malaise, jaundice, amenorrhoea, easy bruising; may mimic acute viral hepatitis.

Signs — jaundice, hepatomegaly, splenomegaly, spider naevi, striae, acne, hirsuties, fluid retention and hepatic encephalopathy may be seen in advanced disease.

Associated disorders

Hashimoto's thyroiditis, Coomb's positive haemolytic anaemia, polyarthritis, vasculitis, lupus erythematosus-like lesions, lymphadenopathy, glomerulonephritis, fibrosing alveolitis, diabetes mellitus, ulcerative colitis, sicca syndrome.

Investigations

1. Full blood count — normochromic normocytic anaemia, neutropenia and thrombocytopenia may occur.
2. ESR raised.
3. Prothrombin time — prolonged, even early in the disease.
4. Liver function tests — serum transaminases are greatly elevated and bilirubin is also raised — levels may fluctuate.
5. Serum globulins — greatly elevated.
6. HBsAg — absent.
7. Serum non-specific antibodies — smooth muscle antibodies (SMA) and antinuclear factor (ANF) are present in 70–80% of cases. Mitochondrial antibodies (AMA) may be present in 30%.
8. Liver biopsy — vital to make diagnosis and to assess if progress to cirrhosis has taken place

Diagnosis

Made if HBsAg is absent, liver histology shows chronic active hepatitis and there is no evidence of other causes of HBsAg negative chronic active hepatitis, especially Wilson's disease and alcoholic liver disease.

Treatment

1. Corticosteroids — with or without an immunosuppressant (e.g. azathioprine) improves symptoms, biochemistry, liver histology and prevents death from liver failure in the short term. Progress to cirrhosis still occurs.
   a. Indications: Not easy to define and depend on clinical judgement but include symptoms, serum transaminases greater than five times upper limit of normal, bridging necrosis on liver biopsy.
   b. Dose: Prednisolone 30 mg/24 h for one week reducing to 10–15 mg/24 h maintenance; continue treatment for six months.
   c. Monitoring of treatment: clinical assessment and liver function tests monthly and repeat liver biopsy at six months.
   d. Remission: occurs when symptoms and biochemistry recover and liver histology improves with loss of inflammatory features. If this occurs, prednisolone is reduced and stopped over two months.
   e. Relapse: indicated by rise in serum transaminases; restart therapy and continue prednisolone for up to three years.
   f. Failure to remit: increase steroids and if no response add azathioprine.

2. Azathioprine — 50–100 mg/24 h; indicated for steroid intolerance or side effects or if no response to prednisolone 20 mg/24 h.
   N.B. Never give it on its own.
3. Cirrhosis — Treat the same as cirrhosis due to other causes.

Prognosis

Greatly improved with corticosteroids and 10 year survival is 60% or greater. Cirrhosis still develops. Varices occur late and causes of death are usually liver failure or bleeding varices.

HBsAg positive chronic active hepatitis

It is commonest in young and middle aged males and more likely in groups at particular risk of hepatitis B infection (see earlier). There is considerable risk of hepatoma.

Clinical features

Presents with chronic hepatitis, unresolved viral hepatitis, advanced chronic liver disease or with the complication of hepatoma. It can be found in asymptomatic HBsAg carriers and discovered because of elevated serum transaminases.

Investigations

1. Liver function tests — moderate elevation of serum bilirubin and transaminases.
2. Serum globulins — moderately elevated.
3. HBsAg — positive.
4. Liver biopsy — shows chronic active hepatitis; orcein bodies (see earlier) and 'ground glass' hepatocytes may be present indicating HBV infection.
5. Hepatoma — should be excluded by measuring α fetoprotein level and by hepatic scanning.

Diagnosis

Demonstration of chronic active hepatitis histologically and HBsAg in serum.

Treatment

1. Corticosteroids — HBsAg positive chronic active hepatitis patients respond less well to steroids than HBsAg negative patients — steroids may actually promote viral replication and continue infectivity. Only symptomatic patients with severe chronic active hepatitis histologically are given steroids; steroid treatment guidelines are the same as in HBsAg negative patients.
2. Antiviral agents, e.g. interferons, adenosine arabinoside-AMP their use is still experimental; early results suggest some transient improvement in liver function with promotion of seroconversion from HBeAg to anti-HBe in some patients.

Prognosis

Slow and insidious course but mild cases can resolve or change to histological picture of chronic persistent hepatitis. Appearance of jaundice is a bad sign indicating a downhill course to liver cell failure, portal hypertension and death. The most serious complication is hepatoma.

CIRRHOSIS

This is a diffuse fibrosis and nodular regeneration of the liver following hepatocellular necrosis; it is defined morphologically.

Causes

Important ones are:

>   Alcohol
>   Viral hepatitis (HBV; non A, non B)
>   Immunological — primary biliary cirrhosis,'autoimmune' chronic
>   active hepatitis
>   Prolonged cholestasis
>   Metabolic, e.g α-l-antitrypsin deficiency, haemochromatosis,
>   Wilson's disease, galactosaemia
>   Drugs and toxins, e.g. methyl dopa, methotrexate
>   Hepatic venous obstruction e.g. Budd–Chiari syndrome,
>   constrictive pericarditis
>   Cryptogenic — heterogeneous group.

Symptoms

Cirrhosis may be asymptomatic and be discovered on routine liver function testing, at laparotomy or at post mortem (compensated cirrhosis). It may present with symptoms of hepatocellular failure i.e. jaundice, fluid retention, hepatic encephalopathy (decompensated cirrhosis) or with complications, e.g. portal hypertension, hepatoma.

Signs

May be none or those of chronic liver disease — e.g. clubbing, leuconychia, palmar erythema, Dupuytren's contractures (alcoholics), spider naevi, telangiectasia (paper money skin), parotid swelling (alcoholics), gynaecomastia, testicular atrophy. The liver and spleen may or may not be palpable. Signs of decompensation are jaundice, bleeding, fluid retention, encephalopathy.

Reason for decompensation

Injudicious use of drugs (especially diuretics, opiates, sedatives), rapid diuresis, dehydration, electrolyte imbalance (especially potassium deficiency), infection, surgery, trauma, gastrointestinal tract haemorrhage.

Investigations

>   **1. Diagnosis of cirrhosis**
>   a. Liver function tests — may be normal in early stages;
>   later bilirubin rises but alkaline phosphatase and serum

transaminases remain normal or are only modestly
elevated
  b. Serum proteins — decreased albumin and raised globulins
     are often the earliest blood abnormalities; however
     proteins may be normal in compensated cirrhosis.
  c. Scanning of liver with ultrasound or radioisotopes
     (technetium) may show features suggestive of cirrhosis
  d. Liver biopsy — only way to make firm diagnosis; may also
     suggest the cause.

2. **Finding the cause**
   The cause may be shown at liver biopsy but often is not;
   minimal investigations are hepatitis markers, serum non-
   specific antibodies (AMA; ANF; SMA), serum ferritin,
   serum α-1 antitrypsin and ultrasound examination to exclude
   large duct biliary obstruction.

3. **Presence of complications**
   a. Portal hypertension — barium swallow and/or upper GI
      endoscopy for varices; portal venography and portal
      venous pressure measurements are indicated if surgery is
      contemplated.
   b. Renal failure and electrolyte imbalance — serum
      electrolytes, urea and creatinine; urine electrolytes.
   c. Hepatic encephalopathy — EEG, daily 'stars' or 'trail
      finding' to assess progress.
   d. Septicaemia or spontaneous bacterial peritonitis — blood
      culture, ascites microscopy and culture (especially if fever
      is present).
   e. Gallstones — pigment stones are common therefore check
      biliary system with ultrasound if levels of bilirubin and
      alkaline phosphatase are greatly elevated suggesting biliary
      obstruction.
   f. Hepatoma — patients with HBV related liver disease and
      haemochromatosis are especially at risk; measure serum α-
      fetoprotein and scan liver using technetium and
      selenomethionine (former is taken up by Kuppfer cells,
      which are not present in hepatoma tissue; latter is taken
      up by normal and malignant hepatocytes).

Treatment

Cirrhosis is irreversible but progression to liver failure and death is not
inevitable, especially if the cause can be removed or minimised (e.g.
stopping alcohol; removing excess iron by venesection; removing excess
copper by chelation). In general:

1. **Compensated cirrhosis**
   a. Remove or minimize the cause.

     b. Advise high protein, high calorie diet; stop alcohol (whatever the cause of the cirrhosis).

     c. Monitor patient regularly for signs of decompensation and for complications.

     d. Check for presence of oesophageal varices.

2. Decompensated cirrhosis

     a. Remove or minimize the cause.

     b. Treat specific aspects of decompensation and problems as they arise (see below).

HEPATOCELLULAR FAILURE

Causes
Virtually any type of liver disease; can be acute or chronic.

Clinical features
General malaise, debility and lethargy, jaundice, fever, fluid retention and ascites, disordered blood coagulation, hepatic encephalopathy, skin changes (spider naevi, etc.), endocrine changes (gynaecomastia, etc.), hyperkinetic circulation, pulmonary changes (hypoxia, cyanosis).

Treatment
The treatment is of the individual aspects of decompensation and of the complications as outlined subsequently.

HEPATIC ENCEPHALOPATHY

It can be acute or chronic.

Causes
Acute or chronic hepatocellular failure; commonest cause of acute encephalopathy is viral hepatitis and of chronic encephalopathy is cirrhosis; chronic encephalopathy may be seen after portasystemic shunts.

Clinical features
Altered sleep pattern, disturbed consciousness, personality change, intellectual deterioration, constructional apraxia, slurred slow speech, flapping tremor (asterixis), fetor hepaticus. In chronic encephalopathy, other neuropsychiatric syndromes may be seen e.g. dementia, fits, cerebellar or basal ganglion disorders. Acute psychiatric states, e.g. hypomania, schizophrenia may occur.

Precipitating factors
Injudicious drug use (diuretics, opiates, sedatives), fluid and electrolyte imbalance as a result of paracentesis, overdiuresis, vomiting, hypokalaemia, gastrointestinal haemorrhage, large protein meal, surgery, alcoholic 'binge', infection, constipation.

Diagnosis and assessment

1. Clinical grading:
   Grade 1 — confused.
   Grade 2 — drowsy.
   Grade 3 — stuperose with marked confusion but obeying simple commands.
   Grade 4 — coma.
   Grade 5 — deep coma with no response to painful stimuli.
2. EEG — marked diffuse changes occur, which may precede clinical signs of encephalopathy. As encephalopathy worsens wave activity becomes less frequent but wave amplitude increases and triphasic activity may occur; in Grade 4 or 5 coma, amplitude lessens and trace may become flat. Similar changes occur with other metabolic encephalopathies e.g. uraemia.
3. Visual evoked responses — are abnormal but their usefulness is currently being assessed.
4. Blood ammonia — levels are raised and usually, but not always, correlate with the severity of the coma. Normal levels are 0.8–1 mg/ml. It is not easy to measure and not required routinely.
5. Clinical assessment — bedside tests for apraxia e.g. 'stars' or 'trail making' test, can be performed daily on the ward or in the clinic to assess progress.

Treatment

1. Identify precipitating causes, if any, and treat.
2. Reduce nitrogen and protein intake — stop all nitrogen containing drugs and stop all dietary protein; give 1500–2000 kilocalories/day, largely as carbohydrate (orally, by nasogastric tube or by i.v. infusion depending on level of coma). As recovery occurs, protein is introduced gradually by 20 g/day carefully assessing response; usually only 40–60 g/day is tolerated.
3. Clear nitrogen from the colon — magnesium sulphate enema once or twice daily while patient is comatose.
4. Minimise production and absorption of nitrogenous substances (e.g. ammonia) produced in the intestine by bacterial metabolism of urea, protein, aminoacids.
   a. Antimicrobials — neomycin 4–6 g orally/day (small risk of hearing or renal damage) or metronidazole 400 mg orally tds; must always be given in severe or acute encephalopathy.
   b. Lactulose — 10–30 ml orally tds particularly useful in chronic encephalopathy; dose may have to be decreased if

there is troublesome diarrhoea; can be given with
antimicrobials.

5. Other treatments if above measures fail — for acute
   encephalopathy L-dopa or i.v. infusion of branched chain
   aminoacids; for chronic encephalopathy L-dopa or
   bromocriptine.

Prognosis

Depends on underlying liver disease.

ASCITES IN CHRONIC HEPATOCELLULAR FAILURE

Clinical features

It can appear suddenly or insidiously and its appearance may be
precipitated by a GI bleed, infection, electrolyte imbalance etc. There is
increasing abdominal girth with dullness in the flanks and shifting
dullness; a fluid thrill is only seen in gross ascites. Increasing intra-
abdominal pressure may precipitate an umbilical, inguinal or incisional
hernia. Marked abdominal swelling contrasts with the wasting and
thinness of the face, chest and limbs. Abdominal striae and dilated
abdominal veins (radiating away from the umbilicus) may be seen.
Associated signs may be pleural effusions, elevated diaphragm, peripheral
oedema. Elevated JVP especially after ascites has been controlled should
suggest a cardiac cause for the ascites.

Investigations

1. Serum urea, creatinine and electrolytes.
2. Urinary electrolytes — collect 24 hour urine sample before
   diuretics have been started; low urinary sodium suggests
   possibility of poor response to treatment.
3. Diagnostic paracentesis — remove 20 ml ascitic fluid for
   microscopy, culture, cytology and protein content. High
   protein content (exudate) can occur in uncomplicated
   hepatocellular failure but should suggest the possibility of
   infection, malignancy or Budd–Chiari syndrome.

Treatment

Initial regime

1. Admit to hospital for bedrest.
2. Restrict salt intake to 22 mmol of sodium/24 h; it is difficult
   for patients to tolerate and excess dietary salt is a common
   reason for 'resistant' ascites.

3. Restrict daily fluid intake to one litre.

4. Give potassium supplements if hypokalaemia is present.

Approximately 20% patients will get a diuresis on these measures especially if it is the first episode of ascites, urinary sodium is greater than 10 mmol/24 h, the liver disease is reversible or ascites has followed infection, bleed, etc.

Diuretics

These are indicated only if the patient has failed to lose weight after 3–4 days on the initial regime. Aim of diuretic therapy is to induce a slow steady diuresis with weight loss of 0.5–1 kg daily. Excessive diuresis may induce encephalopathy and blood volume depletion.

1. Potassium sparing diuretics — initially give amiloride 10 mg/24 h increasing to 20 mg daily; or spironolactone 100 mg daily, increasing to 400 mg daily (risk of gynaecomastia). Both may induce hyperkalaemia therefore reduce dose of any oral potassium supplements.

2. Loop diuretics — use carefully only when potassium sparing diuretics have not induced a diuresis. Start with frusemide 80 mg (or bumetanide 1–2 mg) per day and if no diuresis gradually increase while checking blood urea and electrolytes and check for signs of encephalopathy. Loop diuretics may induce functional renal failure, hyponatraemia, hypokalaemia, hypochloraemic acidosis. The first two imply a poor prognosis. All diuretic therapy must be stopped, at least temporarily, if uraemia or severe electrolyte disturbances develop. Fluid intake is restricted to 500 mg daily, if hyponatraemia develops.

Monitoring of therapy

1. Daily weight and girth measurements.

2. Record fluid intake and output accurately.

3. Blood urea and electrolytes twice a week, or more frequently if derangements are occurring.

Follow-up

After a satisfactory diuresis, the patient is discharged but must be regularly followed up with weight, clinical assessment, blood urea, electrolytes and liver function tests. Diuretics may be reduced and stopped as liver function improves. If patient is well off diuretics, salt restriction can be progressively eased.

Refractory (resistant ascites)

Failure to respond to the above regime suggests poor compliance or severe advanced liver disease with a real risk of functional renal failure and death.

Treatment:

1. Ensure compliance to salt restricted diet and to diuretic medication. If still no response consider (2) and (3) below.

2. Salt poor albumin infusions i.v. — any diuresis may only be

temporary but it may precipitate lasting diuresis in patient whose liver function is beginning to improve.

3. Other measures that may have to be considered in resistant cases:

   a. Ascites reinfusion — either ascitic fluid itself (if sterile) or ultra filtrated ascitic fluid (by means of Rhodiascit machine); it may precipitate a diuresis and allow response to diuretics again in resistant patients.

   b. LeVeen peritoneo–venous shunt — allows continuous ascites reinfusion over many months or even years.

   Both procedures are not without risk and may only work in patients who would respond to diuretic therapy anyway as their liver function improves; however, these procedures may considerably shorten hospital admission time. They have been reported as being helpful in functional renal failure.

4. Contraindicated treatment:

   a. Paracentesis — may precipitate encephalopathy, electrolyte disturbances, volume depletion, circulatory disturbances and renal failure.

   b. Porta–caval shunt — high mortality.

Prognosis

Is that of the underlying liver disease but as ascites is a sign of advanced hepatocellular failure, the prognosis is poor with about 40% 2 year survival.

FUNCTIONAL RENAL FAILURE (Hepato-renal syndrome)

This is renal failure secondary to advanced chronic liver disease and its prognosis is that of the liver disease. It is usually a terminal event and may be precipitated by infection or by plasma volume depletion, e.g. diuresis, paracentesis, diarrhoea, haemorrhage. The main features are refractory ascites with progressive uraemia and/or hyponatraemia.

Treatment

1. Avoid precipitating it by being careful with diuretic therapy
2. Treat any precipitating factor if possible, e.g. infection
3. Stop diuretics and potassium supplements
4. Stop any nephrotoxic drugs, e.g. neomycin
5. Ensure adequate renal blood flow — if necessary by infusion of plasma or salt poor albumin
6. If above fails and patient remains oliguric, restrict all fluids to 500 ml per day.
7. Stop dietary protein

N.B. Renal dialysis does not improve survival and may precipitate GI bleeding and hypotension.

PORTAL HYPERTENSION

This is strictly defined as a rise in pressure in the portal venous system above 7 mmHg. However, it usually refers to the syndrome characterised by the development of porto-systemic anastomoses and splenomegaly. The clinically important portosystemic anastomoses are oesophageal and gastric varices and to a much lesser extent haemorrhoids. Portal hypertension is a factor in the formation of ascites and may be relevant to the occurrence of erosive gastritis in patients with chronic liver disease

Causes

1. Pre-sinusoidal
   a. Intrahepatic — e.g. schistosomiasis, congenital hepatic fibrosis, myeloproliferative disorders.
   b. Extrahepatic — e.g. infection (especially umbilical sepsis), congenital portal vein anomalies, intra-abdominal malignancy, thrombosis following trauma, use of oral contraceptives or associated with enhanced coagulation (as in polycythaemia).
2. Intrahepatic (sinusoidal) — cirrhosis.
3. Post-sinusoidal — e.g. veno–occlusive disease, Budd–Chiari syndrome (hepatic venous or high inferior vena cava block related to malignancy, thrombosis, webs, oral contraceptives, Behçet's syndrome), congestive cardiac failure, constrictive pericarditis.

In patients with pre-sinusoidal portal hypertension, liver function is usually good which is important if shunt surgery is being considered. Patients with intrahepatic or post sinusoidal portal hypertension may go into liver failure if varices bleed.

Clinical features

Portal hypertension may be discovered incidentally or during a search for it in a cirrhotic; it may present insidiously with vague dyspepsia and/or anaemia or acutely with GI blood loss (especially haematemesis) from bleeding oesophageal varices. Important points from the history are any previous episodes of GI haemorrhage or jaundice, drug and alcohol history, haemorrhage, sepsis, abdominal trauma or surgery.

Signs are dilated abdominal wall veins, splenomegaly, ascites or haemorrhoids. Hepatomegaly and the stigmata of chronic liver disease should be looked for. Rectal examination and a faecal occult blood test are necessary.

Investigations

1. Blood tests — full blood count, prothrombin time, liver function tests, urea and electrolytes.
2. Is portal hypertension present?
   a. Indirect — it is indicated by the presence of varices or by the presence of splenomegaly and ascites in a cirrhotic.

b. Direct measurement of portal blood pressure (normal 7 mmHg or less) by direct splenic puncture (the easiest method), at transhepatic venography or by measuring wedged hepatic venous pressure (equivalent to sinusoidal venous pressure).

3. Are varices present?
   a. Barium swallow and/or upper GI endoscopy — the latter may be the better test.
   b. Percutaneous trans-splenic portal venography demonstrates portal vein and varices and is necessary before shunt surgery — it shows whether the portal vein is patent and the portal blood pressure can be measured at the same time. It is contraindicated if coagulation is deranged or if deep jaundice is present.
   c. Coeliac axis angiography — shows portal vein and varices in the venous phase and allows assessment of hepatic artery anatomy which may be helpful to the surgeon. It can be performed in patients with deranged coagulation but portal pressure cannot be measured and injected contrast can precipitate renal failure.

4. Is the portal vein patent?
   a. Ultrasound or CT scanning.
   b. Portal venography — better than indirect scanning.

5. What is the cause of the portal hypertension?
   a. Ultrasound or CT scanning or portal venography will show if portal vein is patent and exclude portal vein obstruction.
   b. Liver biopsy will show intrahepatic disease and the centrilobular congestion of Budd–Chiari syndrome.
   c. Hepatic venography — excludes Budd–Chiari syndrome, webs of the inferior vena cava, etc.

Treatment
None may be necessary if no variceal bleeds have occurred, although prophylactic sclerotherapy of known varices is increasingly being considered. Portal hypertension may cause bleeding varices and their treatment is considered below.

Bleeding Oesophageal Varices

This is the most serious consequence of portal hypertension. Factors leading to variceal rupture are uncertain. Varices may bleed acutely with haematemesis and melaena or chronically resulting in iron deficiency anaemia.

Investigations
Same as in other patients with upper GI haemorrhage (see Ch. 3). Diagnosis is made on upper GI endoscopy which should be done as soon as the patient has been resuscitated, if variceal haemorrhage is suspected.

Treatment

Initial management
This is the same as for any other acute upper GI bleed (see Ch. 9).
Specific points to remember if varices are found and especially if the
patient has evidence of chronic liver disease are:
1. No opiates or strong sedatives. Sedate with a benzodiazepine
   or chlormethiazole if absolutely necessary.
2. Avoid i.v. saline.
3. Check for and correct coagulation deficiencies with vitamin
   K, fresh frozen plasma and platelets as necessary.
4. Give neomycin 1 g orally 4–6 hourly if there are signs of
   encephalopathy after the bleed.
5. Start on H_2 blocker in full dosage as there is a risk of 'stress
   ulceration'.

If the haemorrhage stops
Consider measures to prevent rebleed (see later)

If haemorrhage does not stop spontaneously
1. *Vasopressin* — 20 units in 100 ml 5% dextrose i.v. over 10
   minutes and repeat in a few hours if bleeding continues.
   Alternatively give vasopressin as a continuous i.v. infusion
   (0.4 units/min) for up to 2 hours. Abdominal colic, pallor
   and precipitate defaecation occur and vasopressin is
   contraindicated in patients with ischaemic heart disease.
   Tachyphylaxis occurs. There is no advantage to intra-arterial
   or selective hepatic arterial infusion.
2. *Oesophageal balloon tamponade* (with Minnesota 4 lumen
   tube) — use if bleeding continues despite vasopressin or if
   haemorrhage is torrential. If placed correctly, the tube will
   virtually always arrest haemorrhage. It must be placed by a
   physician skilled in its use. Complications include
   oesophageal perforation and ulceration and aspiration
   pneumonia. The tamponade and traction of the tube are
   maintained for 24 hours (with deflation of the oesophageal
   balloon for a few minutes out of every hour) then both are
   released leaving the tube in situ. If no bleeding occurs, the
   tube is removed but if bleeding restarts, the oesophageal
   balloon is reinflated and traction is maintained for a further
   24 hours. If bleeding restarts again, consider surgery.
3. *Injection sclerotherapy* (see below) can be commenced once
   haemostasis has been secured. The injection may induce
   bleeding which may require a further period of balloon
   tamponade.
4. *Emergency surgery* — reserved for patients who continue to
   bleed or who rapidly rebleed after release of balloon
   tamponade or despite commencing variceal sclerotherapy.
   a. Oesophageal transection — quick, effective procedure in

skilled hands but there is a high mortality; a gastrotomy is required and varices may recur.
   b. Portocaval shunt — high mortality (approximately 50%), particularly in patients with liver failure.

Prevention of rebleed

1. *Injection sclerotherapy* — repeated injections of sclerosant (e.g. ethanolamine oleate) into varices at endoscopy often causes complete obliteration. The number of sclerotherapy sessions varies from one to more than six. Sessions take place at monthly intervals. After obliteration repeated check endoscopies (every six months or so) are necessary to see if varices remain sclerosed. Sclerotherapy reduces the number of rebleeds but may not prolong survival in cirrhotics. It is effective treatment in varices due to non-cirrhotic portal hypertension. Sclerotherapy of gastric varices is not usually possible or successful. Complications include substernal pain, oesophageal perforation, ulceration or stricture, mediastinitis, aspiration pneumonia.

2. *Portasystemic shunt* — various types of surgical shunts have been used, e.g. portocaval, mesocaval, distal spleno-renal. Indications for surgery are definite varices that have bled enough to require transfusion and/or failed sclerotherapy. In cirrhosis there is a high risk of encephalopathy after shunting. The best results are in patients in good nutritional state with no ascites or encephalopathy and with a serum bilirubin $<35\ \mu mol/l$ and a serum albumin $> 35\ g/l$ (Child's group A). Patients with evidence of liver failure (Child's groups B and C) have much worse results. Patients with non-cirrhotic portal hypertension have a much better prognosis after shunting than cirrhotics, but hepatocellular function deteriorates in all patients after shunting and chronic encephalopathy may develop many years after the operation. Careful pre- and post-operative assessment and management is vital with early treatment of liver failure and encephalopathy and avoidance of hepatotoxic drugs and drugs that can precipitate encephalopathy.

3. *Beta blockers* — acutely lower portal venous pressure but there is no evidence of benefit in acute variceal bleeding. There is conflicting evidence as to whether chronic β - blockade decreases rebleeding episodes.

Prognosis

Depends on the effectiveness of the management of a major bleed and the severity of the underlying hepatocellular disease; patients with non-cirrhotic portal hypertension have the best prognosis. Mortality is about 80% in patients with jaundice, ascites and encephalopathy, who have a variceal bleed.

SPACE OCCUPYING LESIONS OF THE LIVER

Causes

1. Carcinoma — by far the most common space occupying lesions in the liver are metastases from primary carcinoma in pancreas, gastrointestinal tract, lung and pelvis. In adults, primary liver cell cancer (hepatoma) is a relatively common termination of cirrhosis, especially in chronic hepatitis B and haemochromatosis, but very rarely occurs in the non-cirrhotic liver.
2. Generalised malignant infiltration of the liver — may complicate Hodgkin's disease, non-Hodgkin's lymphoma and chronic leukaemias and is an occasional feature in highly malignant adenocarcinomas.
3. Benign tumours of the liver are less common but include hepatic adenomas, haemangiomas, hamartomas and a group of odd nodular lesions such as partial nodular transformation.
4. Cysts — may be solitary and large but are commonly multiple and part of the spectrum of polycystic disease; hydatid cysts.
5. Inflammatory space occupying lesions include pyogenic abscess arising de novo or secondary to intraperitoneal inflammation (e.g. diverticular disease, appendicitis). Specific inflammations, such as amoebiasis and tuberculosis, may also cause abscesses in the liver.

Symptoms

These are usually non-specific in the early stages but include anorexia, nausea and weight loss but there may also be symptoms of the primary illness (e.g. colonic carcinoma). Except in inflammatory space occupying lesions and sepsis, pain is an unpredictable feature. It is unusual even in large malignancies, when the growth is relatively slow, but capsular distension by rapidly growing tumours can be distressing.

Signs

Hepatomegaly is virtually always present except in occasional cases where hepatoma arises in shrunken, end-stage, cirrhotic livers. Jaundice and the symptoms and signs of overt liver disease are usually late features. Ascites, although common, is also a late manifestation.

Vascular tumours such as hepatoma or haemangioma occasionally present acutely with abdominal pain, peritonism and shock caused by leak or rupture.

Low grade sustained fevers are very common in hepatic neoplasia but an intermittent high fever is suggestive of an inflammatory lesion.

Supraclavicular lymphadenopathy can sometimes be palpated which then allows diagnosis by fine needle aspiration cytology.

Examination must include careful abdominal palpation for possible primary tumour, subtle ascites, splenomegaly, lymphadenopathy, and a search for evidence of chronic liver disease. Rectal examination and tests for faecal occult blood are essential.

Investigations

Blood tests

1. Liver function tests — space occupying lesions commonly produce marked elevations in the alkaline phosphatase in the absence of clinical biliary obstruction.
2. Alphafetoprotein level — ften raised in secondary neoplasia of the liver and in states of hepatic regeneration but the highest levels are usually seen in hepatoma. When raised, it is a useful means of monitoring progress.
3. Clotting screen — necessary, with platelet count, prior to any invasive diagnostic procedure on the liver.
4. Hepatitis B status — required to assess the necessity for protection of hospital and laboratory staff.

Ascites

If present, aspirate 10–15 ml for microscopy, cytology, culture and protein content. (Protein content not always diagnostically helpful but assists in calculating replacement requirements when therapeutic abdominoparacentesis is necessary)

N.B. Diagnostic cytology of ascitic fluid can be very difficult due to large numbers of other degenerate cells.

Is the space occupying lesion solid or cystic?

Ultrasound scan is best method of detecting cystic lesions. If ultrasound suggests fluid filled or highly vascular lesion, consider abscess, haemangioma, hepatoma. Proceed to hepatic artery angiography, blood cultures or Indium labelled leucocyte scanning as appropriate for clinical picture. Necrotic secondaries often appear cystic but with thick margins of echogenic tissue. Cystic lesions containing crystals, altered blood, etc. can be surprisingly echogenic. If doubt exists, fine needle aspiration of lesion under laparoscopic or ultrasound control is safe in experienced hands in most circumstances except hydatid disease. (Check hydatid compliment fixation test, if this is a realistic differential diagnosis).

Hepatic artery angiography (if appropriate)

Secondary deposits and regenerating nodules take their blood supply mainly from the hepatic artery, not the portal vein. Metastases reveal themselves predominantly as space occupying lesions displacing the vascular architecture. Hepatomas appear as highly vascular lesions in the severely 'pruned' appearance of cirrhotic livers. Haemangiomas are easily diagnosed in livers which are otherwise architecturally normal.

Laparoscopy and liver biopsy

Although the clinical picture and non-invasive assessment (e.g. liver function tests plus ultrasound scan) may indicate a very strong probability of malignant disease, an accurate tissue diagnosis should be obtained in most patients by liver biopsy — some tumours respond well to chemotherapy (e.g. Hodgkin's disease), others may be hormonally sensitive. Laparoscopic liver biopsy is preferable to blind percutaneous biopsy in this situation because:

1. It can ensure that a focal lesion is not missed (e.g. the site of a hepatoma in a cirrhotic liver can often be identified and even minute metastases can be biopsied under direct vision).
2. Inspection of the liver enables better assessment of questionable lesions and avoids indiscriminate puncture of abscesses, haemangiomas, cysts, etc.
3. It enables assessment of complications such as peritoneal involvement, portal hypertension, etc.
4. The procedure is safer than blind percutaneous biopsy in the presence of ascites or clotting deficiency.

Treatment

Malignant deposits

Secondary and primary tumours in the liver are always associated with a bad prognosis and very rarely respond to chemotherapy or radiotherapy. Treatment of the metastases themselves is rarely justified. Similarly, a search for a primary tumour site should only be undertaken if there is a definite indication — e.g. if there is reason to believe the tumour is hormone sensitive (e.g. prostatic carcinoma) or where there is reason to believe the primary is at a site in which it is likely to cause obstruction and palliative bypass may therefore be required. Management is therefore largely symptomatic. Consequently, no specific therapy may be indicated for patients whose hepatic malignancies are asymptomatic, other than emotional and psychological support.

1. *Nutrition* — Anorexia is common and attention should be paid to the maintenance of good nutrition.
2. *Nausea* — is common in advanced lesions and usually responds to treatment with phenothiazines.
3. *Pain* — should be treated with simple analgesics e.g. paracetamol in the first instance, progressing to buprenorphine and traditional opiates as necessary. Avoid analgesic injections if possible — most analgesics have considerably more prolonged action when taken orally.
4. *Malignant ascites* — Treatment is not really indicated unless tense, unpleasantly heavy or painful. Diuretics are disappointing in most cases. Abdominal paracentesis is only effective for short term relief of symptoms but continuous drainage causes severe protein and electrolyte depletion.

Aspirate to dryness and attempt to minimise recurrence using a cytotoxic appropriate for the cell type e.g. 5-fluororacil for GI adenocarcinoma. Intravenous treatment seems as effective as intraperitoneal instillation.

5. *Tumour 'de-bulking'* — Refractory pain, nausea and some other complications (e.g. vena caval compression or obstruction by massive deposits) may require a tumour 'de-bulking' procedure. Probably the best procedure is hepatic artery embolisation via a percutaneous catheter introduced into the appropriate branch(es) of the hepatic artery. This can produce dramatic relief of symptoms in some tumours — noticeably carcinoid tumours, but take care to block the tumours' biologically active secretions using methysergide, cyproheptidine, etc.

Benign tumours

1. *Hamartomas* — usually an accidental finding. Require no treatment.
2. *Solitary cysts* — require no treatment unless causing biliary obstruction when surgical excision is indicated.
3. *Polycystic disease* — assess renal function and treat renal failure and hypertension as appropriate. If a painful cyst can be identified (e.g. after intracystic bleed), aspirate via needle under ultrasound or laparoscopic control.
4. *Haemangiomas* — partial hepatectomy if very large or ruptured.
5. *Adenomas* — stop medication (oral contraceptive, 17-substituted steroids, etc.); regression is then likely.

DRUG-INDUCED LIVER DISEASE

Many drugs influence liver function producing clinically relevant effects but without causing overt liver damage. For example, phenytoin (and many other drugs) induce hepatic microsomal enzymes which influence vitamin D metabolism or concurrent anticoagulant treatment etc.; other drugs interfere at various stages of bilirubin transport to cause jaundice.

However the liver is a major site of metabolism for many drugs which may cause liver injury either acutely or chronically. The hepatic damage may be dose dependent and predictable (i.e. direct hepatotoxic effect) or may in any one individual be unpredictable and independent of dosage (i.e. an idiosyncratic reaction).

Drug-induced liver disease may mimic all varieties of liver disease, but for practical purposes, two main patterns of hepatic damage occur. The clinical picture may be dominated by a pattern of cholestasis (e.g. as occurs with 17-substituted steroids) or by the pattern of hepatitis (e.g. as occurs with halothane). Mixed cholestatic/hepatitic pictures occur (e.g.

with chlorpromazine). Chronic liver disease and cirrhosis may develop insidiously (e.g. with methotrexate) without overt symptoms.

Types of hepatic damage and some causal drugs

1. *Hepatocellular necrosis*
   e.g. Halothane
       Analgesics:
           Paracetamol (in overdose)
           Phenylbutazone
           Indomethacin
           Sulindac
       Sodium valproate
       Methyl dopa
2. *Acute hepatitis*
   e.g. Isoniazid
       Diazepam
       Perhexiline maleate
       Ketaconazole
       Phenothiazines
       Allopurinol
       Monoamine oxidase inhibitors
3. *Chronic active hepatitis*
   e.g. Methyl dopa
       Oxyphenisatin
       Izoniazid
4. *Granulomatous hepatitis*
   e.g. Allopurinol
       Carbamazepine
       Phenytoin
       Penylbutazone
       Hydralazine
5. *Cholestasis*
   e.g. Oral contraceptives & 17-substituted steroids
       Phenothiazines
       Glibenclamide
       Phenytoin
       Carbimazole
       Penicillin
       Erythromycin (estolate)
6. *Cirrhosis*
   e.g. Methotrexate
       Perhexile ne maleate
       Paracetamol
7. *Adenoma and partial nodular transformation*
   e.g. Oral contraceptives and 17-substituted steroids

8. *Veno-occlusive and Budd–Chiari syndromes*
   e.g. Oral contraceptives and 17-substituted steroids
   Mitomycin C
   6-Thioguanine
   Azathioprine

Symptoms and signs may vary from those of fulminant hepatic failure with massive hepatic necrosis, seen in paracetamol overdosage, to minimal or none. Unexplained pyrexia may be a warning sign of hepatic drug sensitivity.

Between the extremes occur relatively mild, nonspecific symptoms such as anorexia or nausea in mild hepatitis or generalised pruritus in mild cholestasis and the more specific illness of clinical hepatitis with typical derangement of liver function tests and obvious cholestatic jaundice and bilirubinuria as described previously.

Most clinical problems arise either because an illness (e.g. pyrexia of obscure origin) may not be recognised as having an hepatic origin or, more commonly, because the liver damage is being caused by a common and usually safe drug which the doctor has failed to recognise as potentially hepatotoxic.

Take a careful history of drug exposure (including over-the-counter drugs) and chemical exposure including occupational history. Examine for signs of acute or chronic liver disease, hepatomegaly, splenomegaly, etc.

Investigations

1. Full blood count — white count is usually normal but eosinophilia may occur in idiosyncratic damage, e.g. halothane.
2. Urinalysis — for bilirubinuria and for urobilinogenuria.
3. Liver function tests
   a. Serum bilirubin — will commonly be raised.
   b. Serum transaminases — raised levels suggest ongoing hepatocellular damage.
   c. Serum alkaline phosphatase — raised levels suggest cholestasis.
   d. Serum proteins — raised globulin or hypoalbuminaemia may indicate chronic liver damage.
4. Serum alphafetoprotein — may be raised in the presence of hepatic regeneration.
5. Clotting screen preparatory to liver biopsy; may be deranged in severe hepatocellular damage.
6. Hepatic imaging — if appropriate in the clinical situation
   a. Ultrasound examination of liver — e.g. to exclude extrahepatic obstruction in patients with cholestasis.
   b. Isotope imaging (selenomethionine scan) — e.g. useful in the diagnosis of veno-occlusive disease and Budd–Chiari syndromes.

    c. Hepatic artery angiography — e.g. if there may be reason
      to expect major vascular abnormalities prior to biopsy.
7. Percutaneous liver biopsy — there is a wide variety of
   possible histological appearances (see above).
8. Withdraw the suspect drug and monitor the effect clinically
   and biochemically. Rechallenge may be appropriate if
   treatment with the putative offending drug is important for
   the patient's health and the hepatic reaction has not been
   severe or life threatening, but caution is required.

Diagnosis

This is always by careful history and liver biopsy, but expert
histopathological interpretation is often required and confirmation of a
drug aetiology may be impossible.
N.B. New hepatotoxic reactions are constantly being reported.

Management

1. Withdraw the offending drug.
2. Inform the patient to prevent re-exposure and record the
   reaction clearly in the notes in a prominent, noticeable
   position. This is particularly important when re-exposure is
   likely to be particularly hazardous, e.g. halothane sensitivity.
   Inform the general practitioner.
3. Correct any side effects resulting from the liver damage, e.g.
   deficiencies of Vitamin D or K resulting from cholestatic
   syndromes, nutritional deficiency, etc.
4. Appropriate symptomatic treatment for hepatocellular failure,
   nausea, pruritus, etc.
5. Specific treatment is rarely required providing the offending
   drug is withdrawn, e.g. chronic active hepatitis may be
   caused by methyl dopa but resolves completely on withdrawal
   of the drug. Established cirrhosis is not influenced by
   corticosteroid treatment which is associated with a high
   incidence of side effects due to decreased steroid metabolism
   in chronic liver disease.

PERCUTANEOUS LIVER BIOPSY

Indications
   Jaundice
   Hepatomegaly
   Unexplained abnormality of liver function

Pyrexia of unknown origin

Suspected hepatitis, cirrhosis, alcoholic liver disease, drug
related disease, reticulosis, intrahepatic malignancy, storage
disease and widespread granulomatous disease

Assessment of response to treatment e.g. chronic active hepatitis

Contraindications

1. *Absolute*
   a. Impaired coagulation — prothrombin time >3 s prolonged
      despite attempted correction; platelet count <80 000/mm^3.
   b. Suspected hydatid cyst, hepatic haemangioma, empyema.
   c. Uncooperative patient.
2. *Relative*
   a. Normal sized liver with normal liver function tests.
   b. Tense ascites.
   N.B. Cholestasis is not a contraindication in the absence of
   infection.

Pre-biopsy tests

Full blood count, prothrombin time, blood group.

Needle

'Menghini' is best for most cases; 'Tru-cut' needle may be useful for hard
fibrous livers.

Procedure

1. Patient is admitted in the morning of the procedure; biopsy
   is only performed when blood results are available.
2. Sedation — normally not necessary.
3. Patient lies flat on back with right hand behind head.
4. The upper border of the liver in the midaxillary line is
   found by percussion. Site of biopsy is usually in area of
   maximum dullness between upper and lower borders.
5. Skin and track between ribs down to liver at right angles to
   skin are anaesthetised with local anaesthetic.
6. Needle is passed to liver surface.
7. Patient breathes out and holds his breath.
8. Needle is rapidly passed into the liver and withdrawn.
9. Patient breathes normally.
10. Liver biopsy is placed on card and immersed in formalin
    solution.
11. Wound is dressed.

If the biopsy has failed, repeat *once* only. Do not attempt biopsy more
than twice at one session.

Post-biopsy care

1. Bed rest 24 h.
2. Pulse and blood pressure regularly for 24 h.

3. Analgesics not usually required but if needed pethidine may be given in small doses.

Reasons for failure

1. Poor technique.
2. Blunt needle.
3. Hard, fibrous or small liver.
4. Ascites.
5. Obesity

Also, sampling errors may occur so lesions missed e.g. tumours, cirrhosis.

Complications

May occur therefore do not perform biopsy late in afternoon or at weekends.

1. Haemorrhage — intrahepatic, intraperitoneal, subcapsular, intrathoracic.
2. Pleurisy.
3. Biliary peritonitis.
4. Haemobilia.
5. Infection, e.g. septicaemia if cholangitis is present.
6. Puncture of other organs e.g. kidney.

Mortality is less than 0.20%.

Alternatives, if coagulation is deranged

1. Percutaneous liver biopsy under cover of fresh frozen plasma and platelet infusions.
2. Percutaneous liver biopsy with 'plugging' of the biopsy hole.
3. Transjugular liver biopsy.
4. Laparoscopic liver biopsy.

13. BILIARY DISEASE

GALLSTONES (CHOLELITHIASIS)

Gallstones are the commonest disorder of the biliary tract.

Composition
Cholesterol, pigment, calcium — 20% are pure cholesterol or pure
pigment stones; 80% are mixed containing at least 50% cholesterol;
10–20% of stones contain enough calcium to be radio-opaque.

Risk Factors

1. For cholesterol stones — increasing age, female sex, obesity,
   oral contraceptives, clofibrate, ileal disease or resection; in
   certain racial groups (e.g. Pima Indians) racial, genetic or
   environmental factors may be important.
2. For pigment stones — chronic haemolysis, cirrhosis of the
   liver.

Clinical Manifestations

1. Acute cholecystitis.
2. Biliary colic and 'chronic cholecystitis'.
3. Obstructive jaundice.
4. Cholangitis.
5. Gallstone ileus (as result of a cholecysto-intestinal fistula
   following episode of acute cholecystitis).

Gallstones are associated with acute pancreatitis and carcinoma of the
gallbladder.
N.B. Probably up to 50% of gallstones are asymptomatic — beware of
ascribing vague dyspeptic or other symptoms to gallstones.

ACUTE CHOLECYSTITIS

This is usually caused by obstruction of the cystic duct by a gallstone.
Bacterial infection is probably a secondary event. Acalculous cholecystitis

is rare but can occur after trauma, surgery, burns or as a complication of typhoid fever, brucellosis, acute pancreatitis, diabetes mellitus.

Clinical features

Biliary 'colic':

1. This is sudden onset, rapidly increasing severe pain situated in the epigastrium and radiating along the right costal margin around to the back under the right scapula.
2. It can sometimes also radiate along the left costal margin as well as occur only on the left or only in the back.
3. It is constant *not* colicky.
4. It often occurs within a few hours of eatiing and at night; it may be associated with nausea and vomiting.

There is often a history of previous episodes of biliary colic, dyspepsia and flatulence.

Signs

Fever, tachycardia, right upper quadrant tenderness and guarding; Murphy's sign may be positive (*N.B.* it is not specific for gallbladder disease); the gallbladder may be palpable and mild jaundice may occur.

Complications

Gallbladder empyema, gangrene or perforation, pericholecystic abscess, hepatic abscess, peritonitis, septicaemia, cholecysto-intestinal fistula.

Investigations

1. Full blood count — neutrophil leucocytosis.
2. Liver function tests — serum bilirubin, alkaline phosphatase and/or transaminases may be raised; bilirubinuria may occur.
3. Blood cultures — may be positive.
4. Plain abdominal radiography — may show gallstones.
5. Ultrasonography — shows gallstones, distended inflamed gallbladder.
6. Biliary scintigraphy — using radiopharmaceuticals (e.g. BIDA) excreted almost exclusively in bile — shows that the cystic duct is obstructed.

Diagnosis

Usually made clinically and confirmed by ultrasound or BIDA scan. Differential diagnosis is from other causes of the acute abdomen (see p. 30) and myocardial infarction (N.B. in cholecystitis and myocardial infarction, serum transaminases can be raised, therefore check serum CPK and ECG to exclude myocardial infarction).

Treatment

1. Pain relief with pethidine or, if the pain is very severe, morphine.
2. Intravenous fluids.
3. Parenteral broad spectrum antibiotics — e.g ampicillin, or a cephalosporin.
4. *Surgery*
   Most cases require surgery unless the patient is very frail

when medical treatment may suffice. Most cases have a cholecystectomy after initial medical treatment; the timing of this is not generally agreed but possibly 2–3 days after the start of medical therapy is best, i.e. during the course of the first admission. Emergency laparotomy is indicated if there is associated peritonitis or if the patient is very ill with an acute abdomen but no definite proof of cholecystitis.

Mucocoele of the gallbladder

The cystic duct is obstructed and the gallbladder becomes filled with mucus; it may be felt as a non tender mass; infection can occur leading to empyema and septicaemia; consideration should be given to cholecystectomy.

Acute emphysematous cholecystitis

The gallbladder wall becomes infected with gas forming organisms so the diagnosis can be made on a plain abdominal radiograph; 20% of patients are diabetic; treatment involves parenteral antibiotics (including cover for anaerobes, e.g. metronidazole) and emergency cholecystectomy. There is a high mortality.

BILIARY COLIC AND 'CHRONIC CHOLECYSTITIS'

Gallstones most frequently present with biliary pain and 'chronic cholecystitis'. There may be attacks of biliary colic (see above) with or without nausea and vomiting and between attacks the patient is well. Alternatively some patients complain of a constant dull ache in the epigastrium or right hypochondrium which may or may not radiate around to the right subscapular region. The only signs may be right upper quadrant tenderness or a positive Murphy's sign. Chronic cholecystitis is a dubious clinical entity although gallbladders removed because of gallstones frequently show histological changes of chronic inflammation. Patients with gallstones frequently complain of flatulence and dyspepsia but these symptoms are common in patients without gallstones and are often not relieved by cholecystectomy.

Investigations

1. Full blood count and liver function tests are normal.
2. Oral cholecystography — confirms the presence of stones; if gallbladder fails to opacify after a double dose of contrast, gallbladder disease can be assumed to be present; cholecystography is mandatory if gallstone dissolution therapy is being considered.

3. Ultrasonography — as good as cholecystography in demonstration of gallstones; allows assessment of bile duct, liver, etc.; useful in pregnant women and in those whose gallbladders fail to opacify at oral cholecystography.
4. Upper gastrointestinal endoscopy — is recommended in those with epigastric pain or dyspepsia to exclude peptic ulcer.

Diagnosis

Gallstones are confirmed by oral cholecystography or ultrasonography; the differential diagnosis of biliary colic includes colonic pain, peptic ulcer, renal and ureteric pain and spinal root pain.

Treatment

Surgery

Cholecystectomy is the treatment of choice in fit patients provided the symptoms are compatible with gallstones; in the frail, elderly or those with severe cardiopulmonary disease, surgery may only be indicated when the symptoms become frequent or intolerable or when complications, (e.g. obstructive jaundice), appear.

Medical therapy

1. *General measures* — weight reduction, low fat diet, analgesics during attacks of pain.
2. *Gallstone dissolution*
   a. Indications — patients unfit for or fearful of surgery; functioning gallbladder on oral cholecystography; radiolucent stones; stones less than 1.5 cm in diameter.
   b. Contraindications — non-functioning gallbladder on oral cholecystography; radio-opaque stones; stones greater than 1.5 cm in diameter; liver disease; females of childbearing age.
   c. Drugs — chenodeoxycholic acid (15 mg/kg/24 h or 20 mg/kg/24 h in the obese) or ursodeoxycholic acid (8-10 mg/kg/24 h).
   Treatment needed for at least six months and often longer. The results depend on stone size — 80% of stones less than 1 cm dissolve in 6 to 12 months and relapse after successful therapy occurs. Response is monitored by oral cholecystography every 2–3 months. Chenodeoxycholic acid can cause diarrhoea and minor liver function abnormality.

Asymptomatic or 'silent' gallstones

There are differing opinions as to whether gallstones found incidentally should be removed or not. The risk of carcinoma of the gallbladder is cited as a major reason for cholecystectomy but the risk is very small.

Only 15% of patients with silent stones go on to develop symptoms and cholecystectomy is not without risk. Therefore, on balance, gallstones should only be removed for *definite* indications. Diabetics may be an exception as they have a much higher morbidity and mortality from acute cholecystitis and emergency biliary surgery than non-diabetics.

GALLSTONES IN THE COMMON BILE DUCT (CHOLEDOCHOLITHIASIS)

Bile duct stones occur in 10% of patients with gallbladder stones. Bile duct stones come from the gallbladder, probably enlarging in the bile duct, or can form de novo in the common bile duct — particularly if there is relative stenosis at the distal end of the duct. They can occur after previous cholecystectomy.

Incidence — increases with age.

Complications — obstructive jaundice, cholangitis, secondary biliary cirrhosis (rare but can occur after long standing biliary obstruction).

Clinical Features

Main symptoms are biliary pain, which is often associated with vomiting, and/or obstructive jaundice which may fluctuate. Painless jaundice may occur; fever is less common and suggests the possiblity of cholangitis.

Signs — none or right upper quadrant tenderness, jaundice or hepatomegaly; the gallbladder is not usually palpable in jaundiced patients i.e. Courvoisier's sign is negative.

Investigations

1. Full blood count — usually normal; neutrophil leucocytosis if cholangitis is present.
2. Liver function tests — normal or serum bilirubin and/or alkaline phosphatase may be elevated if the common bile duct is obstructed; if there is long standing obstruction or cholangitis, serum albumin may be decreased and serum transaminases increased.
3. Prothrombin time — must be checked if percutaneous transhepatic cholangiography or endoscopic sphincterotomy are being considered; may be prolonged if jaundice is present; often correctable with vitamin K.
4. Demonstration of bile duct stones:
   a. Ultrasonography is first investigation and shows whether common bile duct is dilated. It may identify gallstones and demonstrates the state of the gallbladder (if present).
   b. Radiography — intravenous cholangiography (IVC) may

show stones if patient is not jaundiced; however, percutaneous transhepatic cholangiography (PTC) or endoscopic retrograde cholangiopancreatography (ERCP) are preferable especially if the patient is jaundiced (see later).

Diagnosis

Depends on visualisation of the stones; common duct gallstones should be considered in all cases of obstructive jaundice and in patients with biliary pain, especially after cholecystectomy.

Treatment

Aim is to remove gallstones:

1. Exploration of common bile duct via a choledochotomy with removal of stones is the treatment of choice. A transduodenal sphincterotomy may be indicated if a stone is impacted at the distal end of the duct. Stones are easily missed, therefore peroperative cholangiography or choledochoscopy and post-operative T-tube cholangiography are mandatory.
2. Endoscopic sphincterotomy at ERCP is increasingly the treatment of choice in the elderly or frail with bile duct stones; large stones can be removed instrumentally via the sphincterotomy.
3. Retained stones left in the common bile duct after surgery are demonstrated on T-tube cholangiography; they are removed instrumentally via the T-tube track, by perfusion of cholesterol stone dissolving agents (e.g. mono-octanoin) or by endoscopic sphincterotomy; surgery is rarely necessary.

BILIARY TRACT CARCINOMA

Gallbladder

Rare and virtually always associated with gallstones. Usually seen in the elderly presenting with obstructive jaundice, biliary pain or acute cholecystitis. *Diagnosis* is usually made at laparotomy. *Prognosis* is very poor as the tumour is locally invasive and surgery is usually only palliative.

Bile duct (cholangiocarcinoma)

Rarer than gallbladder carcinoma and can occur anywhere in the biliary tree. There is an association with ulcerative colitis. It usually presents with rapidly progressing obstructive jaundice, right upper quadrant pain, hepatomegaly and weight loss — cholangitis is rare. Diagnosed by PTC or ERCP but it can be difficult to separate extrahepatic bile duct carcinoma from benign biliary stricture. Intrahepatic tumour may be diagnosed on liver biopsy. Prognosis is poor and curative surgery is rarely possible but intrahepatic tumour may be successfully treated by hepatic transplant.

CHOLANGITIS

This is bacterial infection in the normally sterile biliary tree; it varies in severity from mild non-suppurative cholangitis to severe acute suppurative cholangitis (with pus in the biliary tree). Partial obstruction as a result of benign strictures or gallstones predisposes to cholangitis. Cholangitis is rarer in complete or malignant obstructions and may be precipitated by biliary surgery, ERCP or PTC.

Organisms — usually enterobacteriaceae especially *E. coli*; mixed growths are common. Gram-positive or anaerobic bacteria are relatively rare.

Clinical features — severe biliary pain, fever, rigors, right upper quadrant tenderness and guarding; tender hepatomegaly may occur and jaundice is often present. Recurrent attacks occur. In acute suppurative cholangitis there is rapid appearance of symptoms and signs and rapid deterioration with features of septicaemia and shock; mental confusion is common especially in the elderly.

Complications — hepatic abscess (often multiple), deterioration of liver function.

Diagnosis — should be suspected if a patient with known or suspected biliary obstruction and/or gallstones becomes ill with fever, rigors, biliary pain and jaundice (Charcot's biliary fever). Diagnosis is confirmed on culture of bile or liver.

Investigations

1. Full blood count — neutrophil leucocytosis (may be absent in elderly).
2. Liver function tests — rapidly worsening with rising serum bilirubin and alkaline phosphatase and falling serum albumin. Serum transaminases usually show a mild rise.
3. Blood cultures — positive; bacteria are also grown from bile or liver biopsy.
4. Definition of obstructing lesion — if biliary tree has not been investigated, ultrasound scan is performed but definitive investigation should wait until the fever, etc. have settled on

antibiotic therapy. In acute suppurative cholangitis there is usually no time for investigation before surgery.

Treatment

 1. *Acute suppurative cholangitis*
 Treatment must be vigorous to prevent rapid deterioration and death.
 a. I.v. fluids; treat shock if necessary.
 b. Antibiotics — do not wait for results of blood cultures, start ampicillin or a cephalosporin with gentamycin i.v.; metronidazole should probably be added as well.
 c. Emergency surgery — this should follow as soon as the patient has been resuscitated. The aim is to relieve the obstruction and drain the biliary tree with the simplest and quickest procedure possible at the time and definitive surgery may have to wait until a second operation. *N.B. The patient is never too ill for surgery because he or she will certainly die without it.*
 2. *Non-suppurative cholangitis*
 a. I.v. fluids if necessary.
 b. Antibiotics.
 The patient usually improves after this allowing investigation. Then treatment is the same as in any other case of extrahepatic biliary obstruction (see — Treatment of 'obstructive jaundice', later in this chapter).

Prevention
Prophylactic antibiotic therapy in all patients with known or suspected biliary obstruction undergoing ERCP, PTC or biliary surgery.

Sclerosing cholangitis

This is a rare condition in which intra- and/or extrahepatic bile ducts are involved in a localised or generalised idiopathic stenosing process; about 50% of cases have ulcerative colitis.

Clinical features — those of cholestasis.

Diagnosis
Liver biopsy and ERCP (or PTC). Liver biopsy appearances can be difficult to distinguish from primary biliary cirrhosis (therefore ERCP should be considered in all cases of PBC). Bile duct appearances, particularly in the localised extrahepatic type of sclerosing cholangitis, can be difficult to distinguish from bile duct carcinoma, therefore diagnostic laparotomy may be necessary.

Treatment
No effective medical treatment. Panproctocolectomy or other treatments for ulcerative colitis do not affect the course of sclerosing cholangitis.

Surgical drainage may be possible for localised extrahepatic disease but hepatic transplant should be considered for advanced cases.

Prognosis

The course is variable and mean survival of fatal cases after diagnosis is 5 years. The usual causes of death are bleeding oesophageal varices or liver failure.

OBSTRUCTIVE JAUNDICE (CHOLESTASIS)

Jaundice is discussed earlier (Ch. 6)

Cholestasis results from obstruction to bile flow anywhere in the biliary tract between the bile canaliculus in the liver and the ampulla of Vater.

Causes

1. *Intrahepatic ('Medical')*
   Cholestatic viral hepatitis
   Drugs; alcohol
   Cirrhosis
   Cholestasis of pregnancy
   Post-operative cholestasis
   Benign recurrent cholestasis
   Primary biliary cirrhosis
   Parasites, e.g. *Clonorchis*

2. *Extrahepatic ('Surgical')*
   Gall stones
   Neoplasia — head of pancreas
                 ampulla of Vater
                 bile duct (also intrahepatic)
                 gall bladder
                 porta hepatis lymph nodes
   Chronic pancreatitis
   Sclerosing cholangitis (also intrahepatic)
   Biliary stricture
   Choledochal cyst

N.B. Patients with cholestasis from one cause (e.g. cirrhosis) may have worsening of their cholestasis due to a second cause (e.g. gallstones). Unrelieved prolonged extra-hepatic biliary obstruction can cause secondary biliary cirrhosis.

Clinical features

Important points from the history are age, foreign travel, abdominal operations, recent injections, recent transfusions, alcohol intake, drugs (including abuse of drugs), previous jaundice, contacts with jaundiced individuals. The typical features of cholestasis are jaundice (which may fluctuate depending on the cause), dark urine, pale stools and pruritus.

As cholestasis progresses without relief, features include steatorrhoea, bone pains, bruising, xanthoma and xanthelasma formation and fluid retention. Fever with jaundice and pain suggests cholangitis; persistent jaundice with progressive weight loss suggests malignancy; jaundice with biliary pain suggests gallstones. The commonest cause of cholestasis in patients under 40 years of age is viral hepatitis and in those over 40 years of age is gallstones.

Signs
These include jaundice, scratch marks on the skin, hepatomegaly, palpable gall bladder (suggests pancreatic carcinoma), palpable mass, stigmata of chronic liver disease, fever (suggests malignancy or cholangitis), splenomegaly (if there is portal hypertension), fluid retention (if there has been hepatic decompensation) and pigmentation, xanthomas or xanthelasma (if cholestasis is long standing).
Rectal examination may show a pale stool (if obstruction is complete) or a 'silver' stool (results from bleeding into the upper bowel in association with cholestasis, e.g. carcinoma of the ampulla).

Investigations

The aim is to confirm obstructive jaundice (cholestasis), determine the level of the obstruction and find the cause.

Confirmation of the diagnosis
1. Clinical features.
2. Urine — contains conjugated bilirubin.
3. Liver function tests — serum conjugated bilirubin and alkaline phosphatase are raised.

N.B. Before proceeding to further investigations, it is necessary in any jaundiced patient to *check*:
1. HBsAg and HBeAg — to exclude hepatitis B infection.
2. Clotting studies — prothrombin time, activated partial thromboplastin time and platelet count.
3. Blood cultures if there is a fever — to exclude infection.

Determination of the level of obstruction
1. Ultrasonography — provides the important information of whether the common bile duct is dilated (suggests extra hepatic biliary obstruction) or not (suggests intrahepatic obstruction); interpretation depends on the skill of the operator and it is easy to miss dilated ducts. It also provides information about liver parenchyma, gall bladder, nodes of the porta hepatis and head of pancreas and may indicate the cause of the obstruction.
2. CT may give the same information but is not indicated, except in elucidating the nature of an abdominal mass in a patient with obstructive jaundice.

Finding the cause of the obstruction

1. If ultrasound suggests dilated ducts, the bile duct must be visualised by one of two approaches:

    a. *Percutaneous transhepatic cholangiography (PTC) with the 'skinny' (or Chiba) needle* — provides excellent views of the bile ducts including the distal common bile duct and it is more likely to be successful than ERCP. It is contraindicated if there is a coagulation defect (same contraindications as for liver biopsy), hypersensitivity to iodinated contrast media, hepatic suppuration or hydatid disease of the liver. There is a risk of bleeding and biliary peritonitis, therefore PTC is contraindicated in patients unfit for surgery. It provides no direct views of the pancreas or ampulla but it can be combined with hypotonic duodenography to investigate the ampulla and pancreatic head. Prophylactic antibiotics should be given if the patient has obstructive jaundice (see later).

    b. *Endoscopic retrograde cholangiopancreatography (ERCP)* — provides good views of the biliary tree as well as the ampulla and allows visualisation of the pancreatic duct. Endoscopic sphincterotomy can be performed at the same time. It is safer than PTC in the frail and in those with coagulation problems. It is more difficult to get satisfactory pictures with ERCP than PTC. The distal bile duct may be less well visualized with ERCP. ERCP is usually not possible in patients with a Polya type partial gastrectomy or with a Roux-en-Y biliary diversion operation. It should not be attempted 4–6 weeks after an attack of acute pancreatitis. Major complications are acute pancreatitis and cholangitis. The risk of the latter is reduced by giving antibiotic cover at ERCP in patients with cholestasis (see later).

2. If ultrasound suggests intrahepatic cholestasis, the following are necessary:

    a. Routine tests for liver disease, e.g. viral studies, serum ferritin, α–1-antitrypsin, etc. (see. 'Investigations' Ch. 6).

    b. Liver biopsy which should suggest the likely cause — if it does not exclude large duct obstruction, PTC or ERCP must be performed.

Treatment

Depends on cause (see elsewhere); aim in all cases is to relieve obstruction if possible.

Surgery for mechanical bile duct obstruction

The aim of surgery is to relieve obstruction and to cure the cause. The procedure performed depends on the cause; often, especially in malignant disease, palliation only is possible by choledochoduodenostomy or by stenting of strictures with external drainage. If the cause is not resectable or the patient is frail, non-operative relief of cholestasis may be done by biliary drainage via the ampulla of Vater (catheter inserted at ERCP) or by passage of stents percutaneously through the liver. Such techniques may be used to relieve cholestasis before definitive and curative surgery (e.g. resection of the pancreatic head) as the results of surgery may be improved.

Surgery in jaundiced patients
These patients are poor risk subjects for major surgery. Prognosis can be improved by:
1. Vitamin K 10 mg i.v. daily for three days pre-operatively.
2. Parenteral or enteral nutrition for two weeks pre-operatively, if it is safe to delay surgery and if the patient is malnourished and hypoproteinaemic.
3. Prophylactic antibiotics — for 24 hours pre-operatively or single dose per-operatively; choice depends on local bacterial sensitivities (usual choices are ampicillin or a cephalosporin with gentamicin if the patient is ill).
4. Pre-operative biliary drainage (see above).
5. Prevention of acute renal failure — patients with cholestasis (especially if bilirubin is greater than 170 μmol/l) are at risk of post-operative acute tubular necrosis. It may also occur after ERCP or PTC. It is often precipitated by prolonged (> two hour) hypotension (systolic BP < 90 mmHg).

Prevention — prophylactic antibiotics; good hydration pre-operatively; mannitol 10% 200 ml i.v. per-operatively, which is repeated if urine output falls below 60 ml/h. Pre-operative biliary drainage may reduce incidence of renal failure.

Treatment of protracted cholestasis

Unrelieved cholestasis causes:
1. **Pruritus** — treat with cholestyramine 4 g/24 h increasing to 16 g/24 h if necessary; very often not tolerated by the patient and the alternative is aluminium hydroxide gel.
2. **Malabsorption of**:
   a. Vitamin K causing prolonged prothrombin time and bruising — treat with vitamin K 10 mg oral/24 h.
   b. Fat causing steatorrhoea — low fat diet (40 g/24 h).
   c. Vitamin D and calcium causing osteomalacia and osteoporosis — vitamin D (e.g. calciferol 150 000 units weekly) or vitamin D analogues (e.g. alfacalcidol 1 microgram daily); calcium 40 mmol/24 h as effervescent calcium one tablet qds.
   N.B. Do not give at the same time as cholestyramine as the latter binds calcium.

3. **Hypercholesterolaemia** — which results in xanthomas and xanthelasmas. No treatment is required except if xanthomatous neuropathy occurs, which can be relieved by plasmapheresis.

PART THREE
Nutritional support in gastro-intestinal disease

14. MALNUTRITION

Malnutrition is particularly common in diseases of the gastrointestinal tract. Hospital surveys in Western countries have revealed a high prevalence of malnutrition in medical and surgical patients. An appreciation of its causes and potential consequences is fundamental to the assessment of nutritional status and the provision of nutritional support. Once a decision to provide nutritional support has been made, key questions must be asked to ensure that the correct route is chosen. Certain conditions, such as liver disease, necessitate individual consideration to avoid complications.

Table 14.1 Causes of malnutrition in gastrointestinal disease

Causes of malnutrition	Example of clinical condition
Reduced intake	
Poor diet	alcoholism
Anorexia	carcinoma
Taste disturbance	carcinoma, zinc deficiency
Fear of eating (pain)	peptic ulcer, Crohn's disease
Poor mastication	poorly fitting dentures, oropharyngeal carcinoma
Dysphagia	
mechanical	carcinoma of oesophagus stricture
neuromuscular	achalasia, progressive systemic sclerosis
Early satiety	post-gastrectomy
Vomiting	pyloric stenosis
Reduced absorption	
Maldigestion	
biliary	obstructive jaundice
pancreatic	carcinoma of pancreas, chronic pancreatitis
inactivation of digestive juices	Zollinger–Ellison syndrome
Binding of nutrients in lumen of bowel	phytate excess — binds some minerals
Mucosal disease	coeliac disease, Crohn's disease
Bacterial overgrowth	surgical blind loop, Crohn's disease, progressive systemic sclerosis
Fistulation	Crohn's disease,
Poor motility	Intestinal pseudo-obstruction
Major bowel resection	Crohn's disease, mesenteric
(Short bowel syndrome)	vascular thrombosis
Excess losses	
Hypercatabolism	fulminant ulcerative colitis, post-operative states
Protein losing enteropathy	gastric carcinoma, inflammatory bowel disease

ASSESSMENT OF NUTRITIONAL STATUS

An awareness of possible malnutrition is a key factor in clinical assessment. There is no one diagnostic test — history and examination are important and can be backed up by biochemical, haematological and immunological investigation.

History
Duration of illness, weight loss, knowledge of previous healthy weight, dietary intake assessment.

Examination
Apathy, emaciation, lax wrinkled skin, muscle wasting and weakness, dry falling hair, dependent oedema, angular stomatitis, anaemia. These are all signs of severe malnutrition. There may be no physical signs other than weight loss. Beware the presence of oedema which may mask weight loss.

Anthropometry

1. *Weight* — can be expressed as percentage of ideal weight[a] or, better, used to calculate the Quetelet Index (QI).

   $$QI = \frac{\text{Weight (kg)}}{\text{Height}^2 \text{ (m}^2\text{)}}$$

   Normal: Men 20.1–25.0
   Women 18.7–23.8

2. *Mid-arm circumference* (MAC) — circumference of non-dominant upper arm measured midway between acromion and olecranon.

3. *Triceps skin fold thickness* (TSF) — use calipers to measure thickness of skin and subcutaneous tissue pulled gently away from triceps muscle.

4. *Mid-arm muscle circumference* (MAMC) — calculated, using formula:

   $$MAMC = MAC - (\pi \times TSF)$$

5. *Biceps skinfold* — at same level as triceps, over biceps muscle.

6. *Subscapular skinfold* — measured just below left scapula along plane of dermatome.

7. *Suprailiac skinfold* — above left superior iliac crest in mid-axillary line.

Table 14.2 Values suggestive of protein energy malnutrition

Weight loss	> 10% normal weight	
	Male	*Female*
MAMC[b]	< 20.2	< 18.6 mm
TSF[b]	< 10	< 13.2 mm
Sum of four skinfolds	<40 mm	

[a] *See* Jelliffe D B 1966 The Assessment of the Nutritional Status of the Community. World Health Organisation, Geneva
[b] Values given are 80% standard measurements

Biochemical investigations

1. *Serum albumin* measurements provide useful information about the patient's nutritional state in the absence of parenchymal liver disease or proteinuria. Because of its long half-life it is a poor monitor of response to nutritional support.
2. *Serum transferrin* has a more rapid turnover but its usefulness is limited in the presence of iron deficiency where levels are high.
3. *Thyroxine-binding pre-albumin* and *retinol binding protein* serum levels are reduced in protein energy malnutrition and because of their short half-lives and rapid turnover are quick to respond to improvements in nutritional status.
4. Look for specific deficiencies of *vitamins, trace elements, calcium, iron* etc. and it is more important that the composition of the nutritional support instituted includes adequate amounts of these nutrients to fulful requirements.

Immunological tests

1. Protein energy malnutrition is associated with impaired immunocompetence.
2. The peripheral blood lymphocyte count is reduced and increases with nutritional support.
3. Impaired delayed-hypersensitivity reactions to common antigens can be identified by skin testing. A negative reaction is induration less than 5 mm in diameter 48 hours after intradermal injection. Reversal of this immunological anergy may be seen after nutritional support.
4. Use of *Candida albicans* antigen alone is suitable for clinical practice.

Table 14.3 Values suggestive of protein energy malnutrition

Serum albumin	< 35 g/l
Serum transferrin	< 2g/l
Serum pre-albumin	<100 mg/l
Serum retinol binding protein	<30 mg/l
Lymphocyte count	< 1 × 10⁹/l
Candida albicans antigen 0.1 ml 1 in 100 dilution	< 5 mm induration

INDICATIONS FOR NUTRITIONAL SUPPORT AND SELECTION OF ROUTE

Indications

1. *Gross malnutrition* — with obvious hypoproteinaemic oedema, muscle wasting and weight loss.
2. *Probable malnutrition* — with anthropometric, biochemical

and immunological indices suggestive of protein-energy
malnutrition. A history of poor dietary intake and weight loss
is helpful.

3. *Potential malnutrition* — where the patient has developed
anorexia, dysphagia, a catabolic illness or some other
condition which will result in impaired oral intake.

4. *Bowel rest* — in some conditions, for example Crohn's
disease, a decision to specifically prohibit oral or enteral
intake will require nutritional support via an alternative
route.

Route of administration

1. *Oral*: provided no obstruction to access — anorexic,
neurological or mechanical — to a functioning gastrointestinal
tract. In practice use only in cases of mild nutritional
depletion. Otherwise opt for:

2. *Enteral*: using fine bore nasogastric catheter (or sometimes
post-operatively via gastrostomy, duodenostomy or
jejunostomy). Use in preference to parenteral route if at all
possible. Ask the following questions:
   a. *Is the gastrointestinal tract accessible?*
      Most oesophageal carcinomas do not obstruct the lumen
      entirely. Fine bore catheters can be passed endoscopically.
   b. *Is the gastrointestinal tract functional?*
      Even in cases of small intestinal disease, enough digestive
      and absorptive capacity remains for effective enteral
      nutrition in many cases.
   c. *Will the maximum tolerated gastrointestinal intake be
      sufficient?*
      In catabolic states it may be necessary to use parenteral
      nutrition simply because it is possible to administer greater
      amounts of nitrogen and energy this way.

3. *Parenteral*: use this route only if it is not possible to provide
satisfactory nutritional support via the enteral route.

NUTRITIONAL REQUIREMENTS

1. **Energy**
   Minimum requirement during illness is 30 kcal/kg/24 h,
   rising, in states of moderate catabolism (such as post-op
   with infection) to 45 kcal/kg/24 h and, in severe catabolic
   states (trauma, burns) to 67 kcal/kg/24 h.

2. **Nitrogen**
   For most hospitalised, not excessively catabolic patients,
   give according to a non-protein energy (kcal) to nitrogen (g)
   ratio of 200:1, or in catabolic patients 150:1. Nitrogen

provision can be adjusted by estimating nitrogen balance
from a 24 hour urine collection.

3. **Fat**
   Give 500 ml 10% 'Intralipid' weekly to satisfy essential fatty
   acid requirements. In patients with only modest energy
   expenditure and nitrogen requirements approximately half
   the calories can be given in the form of fat (and half as
   glucose). Many authorities prefer to avoid giving much fat
   to excessively catabolic patients.

4. **Water**
   Normal requirement is approximately 30 ml/kg/24 h or
   1 ml/kcal, increasing in fever, catabolic states and with
   abnormal losses.

5. **Sodium**
   Depends on clinical situation with high requirements for
   patients with fistula losses, and low requirements in renal or
   liver disease.

6. **Potassium**
   Give at least 5 mmol K^+ with each gram of nitrogen and
   greater amounts when there is a pre-existing deficit, in
   patients who are anabolising, and in those receiving glucose
   and insulin.

7. **Phosphate**
   An important constituent especially in parenteral nutrition.
   Give a minimum of 0.5 mmol/kg\24 h. The phosphate
   present in 'Intralipid' may not be 'available'.

8. **Magnesium**
   Magnesium deficiency is relatively common particularly from
   intestinal fluid loss and diuretic therapy. Give 5 mmol/24 h,
   but up to 15 mmol/24 h may be needed when there are
   excessive gastrointestinal losses.

9. **Calcium**
   Calcium supplements are unnecessary for feeding periods of
   less than two weeks. For longer periods give
   0.1 mmol/kg/24 h.

10. **Zinc**
    Plasma levels are not a good guide to requirements unless
    they drop very low. Give 50–200 μmol/24 h.

11. **Iron**
    Daily requirement is 20–70 μmol/24 h.

12. **Other trace elements**
    Deficiencies of chromium, selenium, copper and
    molybdenum may occur with prolonged feeding.

13. **Vitamins**
    Most patients receiving parenteral nutrition need more than
    the recommended daily allowances.

15. ENTERAL NUTRITION

Enteral feeding can be given in addition to continued oral intake, as the sole nutritional intake, or with intravenous nutrition as the latter is tailed off.

1. **Catheter**
   Use a fine bore tube passed into the stomach. Check for correct catheter position by auscultating over the abdomen while injecting air or taking a chest and upper abdominal X-ray. Endoscopic placement is sometimes necessary especially when passage to the duodenum is required.

2. **Pump**
   If available use a pump as the rate of infusion can be better controlled and the catheter is less likely to block. Purpose built enteral feeding pumps are reliable and relatively cheap.

3. **Reservoir**
   Drip feeding is much more satisfactory than bolus feeding. Use a reservoir; some are supplied with inbuilt infusion sets. Fill every six hours and replace every 24 hours. Infuse for 18 out of 24 hours; discontinue feeding during the night in elderly patients (risk of aspiration) and during the afternoon in younger ambulant patients.

SELECTION OF ENTERAL DIET

Hospital-prepared liquid diets

Advantages — relatively cheap (but the cost of the diet–kitchen facility must be considered) and can be tailored to patients' needs but are outweighed by *disadvantages* (non-sterile; usually milk-based; full trace element and vitamin composition probably not known, increased incidence of diarrhoea).

158

Proprietary whole–protein diets

These should be used in preference to elemental diets, which are more expensive and should be reserved for specific indications. Consider the following:

1. **Nutritional completeness** — all essential nutrients should be present in sufficient quantities at least to meet the Recommended Dietary Allowances.
2. **Osmolality** — use a diet which at full strength is less than 400 mosm/kg.
3. **Energy/nitrogen ratio** — for the moderately catabolic patients this should be (kcal/gN) approximately 200:1. For greater degrees of catabolism 150:1 may be more appropriate. Although this ratio can be adjusted by the addition of a glucose polymer solution such as 'Caloreen', this will impair the sterility of the diet.
4. **Lactose and gluten** — use a gluten-free diet in coeliac disease. Lactose intolerance is common among Asians, Africans and Southern Europeans and may temporarily occur in gastrointestinal disorders in others. In these circumstances use a lactose-free preparation.

Chemically-defined 'elemental' diets.

These diets are composed of small peptides and amino acids, and glucose as the energy source. Their availability before the cheaper whole protein preparations has led to their use in inappropriate situations. In general their use should be reserved for:

1. **Impaired digestion**: disorders of exocrine pancreas, short bowel syndrome.
2. **Reduced absorptive capacity**: intestinal resections and fistulae, severe untreated coeliac disease.
3. **Crohn's disease**: recent evidence suggests a beneficial effect on active disease.

ADMINISTRATION

Pump-controlled continuous infusion through fine-bore catheters has reduced the necessity for 'starter diets' particularly for whole protein diets of osmolality less then 400 mosmol/kg. Higher osmolality elemental diets may require a 'starter diet' with gradual increments of volume and concentration over three to four days.

COMPLICATIONS OF ENTERAL NUTRITION

Tube related complications

The use of flexible, fine-bore feeding tubes has effectively eliminated the problems of oesophageal ulceration, haemorrhage and stricture–formation previously associated with the larger more rigid Ryles tubes.

Misplacement of the tube into the trachea and subsequent infusion can be avoided by always checking that the tube is in stomach.

Aspiration

Much less frequent with fine-bore tubes which do not interfere with anti-reflux mechanisms. Elderly, obtunded and unconscious patients are most at risk. The hazard can be minimized by slow pump-controlled feeding, raising the head of the bed, administering the diet into the jejunum or discontinuing the feed during the night.

Gastrointestinal side-effects

Nausea, vomiting, abdominal cramps and distension are usually minor problems that can be alleviated by a reduction in the rate of infusion. Diarrhoea is rarely troublesome even with the high osmolalities of elemental diets. When it does occur other factors such as concurrent antibiotic therapy, lactose intolerance, or bacterial contamination of the enteral feed should be considered.

Metabolic complications

Hyperglycaemia, especially in catabolic patients with a relative insulin lack, and electrolyte problems may occur.

Liver function abnormalities

Elevation of hepatocellular enzymes, alkaline phosphatase or bilirubin may occur; the aetiology is uncertain.

Nutritional problems

Most proprietary enteric preparations are nutritionally satisfactory, but many anabolic patients will have increased requirements for zinc and potassium. Some elemental diets have very little fat and essential fatty acid deficiency may result.

16. PARENTERAL NUTRITION

The basis of all indications for parenteral nutrition with the exception of the provision of bowel rest, is the inability to provide satisfactory nutritional support via the gastrointestinal tract.

1. **Catheter**

   Those made out of silicone elastomer are less irritant to the vein. Insertion, under aseptic conditions should be into a central vein, preferably the subclavian vein approached via the infraclavicular route. A skin tunnel prolongs catheter life by reducing the risk of infection and enabling the catheter to be fixed more securely. Confirmation of intravascular placement is made by allowing backflow of blood by lowering the infusion bag below the level of the heart. The position of the catheter tip which should be in the superior vena cava is checked by penetrated chest X-ray.

2. **Dressing**

   After insertion the catheter entry and skin tunnel exit sites are sprayed with iodine. A semipermeable transparent adhesive dressing is then applied and only changed if there are signs of sepsis.

3. **Pump**

   Control of the infusions is made safer and simpler by the use of pumps equipped with an alarm system. These are expensive and prevention of inadvertent rapid infusion can be avoided by use of a biurette.

4. **Once daily bag system**

   Mixture, under sterile conditions, of all the nutrients required for parenteral nutrition (glucose, amino-acids, fat emulsion, trace elements, vitamins and minerals) obviates the need for changing bottles on the ward, and reduces the risk of infection.

SELECTION OF PARENTERAL NUTRITION SOLUTIONS

As in enteral feeding, nutritional requirements consist of an adequate balance of nitrogen and energy supplemented by trace elements, vitamins and electrolytes.

1. **Nitrogen**

   Synthetic L-amino acid solutions containing both essential and non-essential amino acids have replaced the previously available protein hydrolysates. There is discussion over the theoretical advantages and disadvantages of the various commercially available solutions but particular clinical advantages of one over another have not been demonstrated. In practice it is better for the clinician to familiarise himself with a small number of preparations.

2. **Energy:** *Glucose*

   This is the carbohydrate of choice — all tissues metabolise glucose. In catabolic patients, problems with insulin resistance and hyperglycaemia can normally be overcome by an infusion of exogenous insulin. Reactive hypoglycaemia may follow infusion of 50% glucose after such concentrated solutions. In practice the use of the once daily bag eliminates this potential problem.

   Fructose, sorbitol, ethanol

   Metabolic problems, lactic acidosis or toxic effects far outweigh any potential advantages.

   Fat

   Advantages: high calorific value, isotonic, prevents essential fatty acid deficiency, vehicle for fat soluble vitamins. Used in conjunction with carbohydrate it has a nitrogen sparing effect and is a useful source of energy in moderately catabolic patients. In septic hypercatabolic patients it has been customary to avoid fat but recent evidence suggests this is not necessary. Fat emulsion can be mixed with other nutrients in a once daily bag system.

3. **Vitamins and minerals**

   Daily requirements are impossible to predict with certainty. Regular use of proprietary vitamins and trace element supplements, regular biochemical monitoring and strong clinical awareness of potential for deficiencies will prevent problems. Particular awareness required for folate — utilised rapidly in an anabolic patient receiving amino acids; deficiency leads to leucopenia, thrombocytopenia and anaemia; *zinc* — involved in the metabolism of over 100 enzymes; *phosphate* — requirements not known with accuracy but supply should be guided by regular serum phosphate measurements.

DESIGNING A REGIMEN

1. *Ill patients* — such as renal failure, severe trauma, sepsis or gross electrolyte upset may need daily adjustments to their prescription depending on results of biochemical monitoring.

2. *Stable, less catabolic patients* — can usually be given a standard regimen repeated every 24 hours.

3. *In theory* — detailed assessment of the individual patient and calculation of metabolic needs (see under Nutritional Requirements) should be performed.

4. *In practice* — the availability of one or two standard regimens in a hospital will meet the needs of the majority of patients.

Table 16.1 Example of regimen using once-daily bag system

Vamin glucose	1500 ml
Glucose 20%	1000 ml
Intralipid 20%	500 ml
Addamel	10 ml
Potassium phosphate solution	30 ml
Vitlipid	10 ml
Solivito	1 vial
	3050 mls

This regimen provides:

Nitrogen	14.1	g
Energy (non-protein)	2775	kcal
Glucose	350	g
Fat	100	g
Sodium	90	mmol
Potassium	85	mmol
[a]Magnesium	3.1	mmol
Phosphate	35.5	mmol
[a]Zinc	20	μmol

[a] Further zinc and magnesium supplementation may be necessary

COMPLICATIONS OF PARENTERAL NUTRITION

Catheter related problems:

1. Pneumothorax — experienced operator required.
2. Air embolism — patient should be in head down position.
3. Haemothorax, arterial puncture, nerve injury.
4. Superior vena cava thrombosis (rare) — may avoid by infusing low dose heparin (1000 units/day) with nutrients.

5. Sepsis
   a. Carefully kept temperature chart is mandatory.
   b. Other sources of infection should be excluded.
   c. Catheter entry site is swabbed, and catheter removed if no other source is apparent.
   d. If pyrexia continues and positive blood cultures obtained antibiotics are instituted.

Metabolic complications

1. Hyperglycaemia
2. Glycosuria and osmotic diuresis
3. Hyperosmolar non-ketotic coma
} Known diabetic and hypercatabolic patients most at risk. Careful monitoring and correction with insulin infusion required.

4. Reactive hypoglycaemia — Avoid by always following 50% glucose with more dilute glucose solution.
5. Lactic acidosis — At risk with fructose, sorbitol or excess amino acids.
6. Nutritional deficiencies (especially during anabolism) — Folic acid, zinc, potassium, magnesium, phosphate.

Liver function test abnormalities

1. Cholestasis — thought to be due to biliary sludge.
2. Raised transaminases — May be due to fatty liver, either from pre-existing malnutrition or from use of excessive energy supplies.
3. Hepatic dysfunction, other than due to parenteral nutrition, may be responsible.

MONITORING

Purpose

1. Early detection of metabolic complications.
2. Detection of deficiency states.
3. To record nutritional response of the patient.

Observations and investigations

Daily

Fluid balance and temperature
Serum urea and electrolytes (twice weekly when stable)

        Blood glucose (several times if unstable)
        Urinalysis for glycosuria (4 hourly)
Twice weekly
        Body weight
        Full blood count including platelets
        Liver function tests and prothrombin time
        Serum calcium, phosphate
Once weekly
        Anthropometric measurements
        Lymphocyte count
        Serum proteins
        Serum zinc, copper, magnesium, iron
        Serum vitamin B_{12}
        Serum folate
        24 hour urinary urea

Nitrogen balance
Weekly estimation of nitrogen balance is useful to ensure adequacy of
the regimen and can be calculated from the 24 hour urinary urea
excretion on the basis of the following assumptions:
        1. Faecal nitrogen excretion is fairly constant at 1–2 g daily in
            the absence of diarrhoea even in severe catabolic illnesses
        2. The majority of nitrogen in urine is present as urea.
Nitrogen excretion (g) = (urine urea [mmol/24 h] $\times$ 0.034) + 2.

17. NUTRITIONAL ASPECTS OF LIVER DISEASE

Patients with cirrhosis are frequently malnourished because of poor intake, decreased absorption, metabolic and hepatic storage abnormalities. There are pitfalls in standard nutritional assessment:

> Weight loss — may be masked by oedema and ascites
> Immunological anergy — may be due to factors other than protein energy malnutrition
> Reduced visceral protein levels — may result from reduced hepatic synthesis.

Nutritional support in the absence of hepatic encephalopathy

Standard enteral and parenteral products should be used unless deterioration occurs. Many patients with hepatic cirrhosis are erroneously treated with a low protein diet in the absence of encephalopathy.

Nutritional support in encephalopathic patients

These patients will deteriorate if given standard formulations and yet will become more malnourished if treated by standard means with protein restriction.

Recent work suggests that enteral and parenteral products rich in branched chain amino acids (BCAA) and low in aromatic amino acids (AAA) (which complement the disordered BCAA : AAA ratio found in these patients) may be nutritionally beneficial without causing deterioration in hepatic encephalopathy. Whether they specifically improve the encephalopathy has not yet been established.

FURTHER READING

Bateson M C, Bouchier A D 1981 Clinical investigation of gastrointestinal function. Blackwell, Oxford
Bouchier A D, Allan R N, Hodgson H J F, Keighley M R B 1984 Textbook of gastroenterology. Ballière Tindall, London
Shearman D J C, Finlayson N D C 1982 Diseases of the gastrointestinal tract and liver. Churchill Livingstone, Edinburgh
Sherlock S 1986 Diseases of the liver. 7th edn. Blackwell, Oxford
Silk D B A 1983 Nutritional support in hospital practice. Blackwell, Oxford
Sleisenger M H, Fordtran J S 1983 Gastrointestinal disease. 3rd edn. Saunders, Philadelphia

INDEX